RELAXED & READY

A SIMPLE ROADMAP
TO REDUCING WORKPLACE
STRESS AND FRUSTRATION

RELAXED & READY

Deitrick L. Gorman, DO

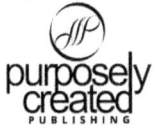

RELAXED AND READY
Published by Purposely Created Publishing Group™
Copyright © 2019 Deitrick L. Gorman

All rights reserved.

No part of this book may be reproduced, distributed or transmitted in any form by any means, graphic, electronic, or mechanical, including photocopy, recording, taping, or by any information storage or retrieval system, without permission in writing from the publisher, except in the case of reprints in the context of reviews, quotes, or references.

Printed in the United States of America

ISBN: 978-1-64484-024-5

Special discounts are available on bulk quantity purchases by book clubs, associations and special interest groups.
For details email: sales@publishyourgift.com or call (888) 949-6228.
For information log on to: www.PublishYourGift.com

DISCLAIMER

Please note that I am fully aware that our human body, in my opinion, is awesome and beautifully designed. It is also very complex and integrated on many levels. It is actually quite mind boggling, if you really think about it. Plus, researchers are discovering new ways our body works. Having said that, please don't be upset that I did not discuss every single function of the hormones or every single intricacy of muscles mentioned in this book. They are discussed for the purposes of basic understanding. For more in-depth understanding, I invite you to take classes or purchase necessary books. Thanks!

*To my mama, Gladys, simply . . .
thank you for it ALL.*

*To my fiancé, Kasaly, thank you, honey,
for your love and support.*

*To my sisters, Letha Rae and Katrina,
thanks for believing in me.*

*To my work family at Reeves County Hospital,
thank you for your acceptance and support.*

*I would like to dedicate my first book to those
people who know there is a better way to handle*

*their stress at work but are not sure what it is.
You are not alone. I've been there. Don't lose hope.*

TABLE OF CONTENTS

Introduction 1

CHAPTER 1:
Evaluating the Cause of Your Stress at Work 13

CHAPTER 2:
Toxic Work Environments 25

CHAPTER 3:
Dealing with Challenging Coworkers 33

CHAPTER 4:
Stress Can Affect You Physically, Chemically,
Hormonally, Mentally, Emotionally, and Behaviorally ... 47

CHAPTER 5:
What Unmanaged Stress Does to You at Work 65

CHAPTER 6:
Benefits of Relaxation at Work 73

CHAPTER 7:
Relaxation Hormones 81

CHAPTER 8:
How to Manage Stress at Work 89

CHAPTER 9:
Mindful Relaxation at Work 103

CHAPTER 10:
Declutter Your Office Space 117

CHAPTER 11:
Zen Your Work Space 127

CHAPTER 12:
Self-Care 135

BONUS:
Work Stress Action Plan 147

BONUS:
A Message to Company Heads, Business Owners,
Managers, and Bosses 155

BONUS:
Color Now (3 pages of Coloring) 165

BONUS:
30 Days of Calm (A 30 Day Interactive to Help You
Destress at Work) 169

About the Author 183

INTRODUCTION

What is stress? Stress is an externally applied force. Stress can be external or internal. An example of external stress is weight lifting. When you lift weights, you are using these weights to "stress" your muscles so that these muscles can change and become stronger and sometimes bigger to accommodate that extra weight.

An example of an internal stress is needing to meet a deadline. Worry is also an internal stress.

Stress isn't always a bad thing. It can be good or in fact great—but only in the short term. It can help us perform better physically and mentally by having us "rise to the occasion." Short-term stress can aid us in fleeing a dangerous situation or giving us the brief time to focus and perform well. In the work setting, stress can help us meet a deadline or deliver an amazing presentation.

In the long term, however uncontrolled chronic stress can be detrimental to your personal health, family interactions, and job performance.

If we look at the weight lifting example, when an external force is applied to your muscles (lifting the weights), as you gradually add extra pounds to the weights over time, those muscles get stronger and bigger. But if you were to go to the gym today and immediately try to lift a very heavy weight that you have never tried to lift, you can damage your muscles.

It's not exactly the same thing with that internal stress. In the short term, it can be beneficial, but having constant, chronic mental stress can actually tear you down. This can affect you in many different ways. In the work setting, you become nonproductive, disengaged, cranky, and unfocused. This is not to mention what chronic stress does to your overall health. We will talk about that.

Unless you have hit the lottery or inherited a big chunk of money and managed your money appropriately such that you never have to work again, we all have to go to work. Whether you have undertaken the aspiration to start your own business or you are working for an employer, you will at some point experience stress. Heck, even if you are already wealthy, I'm sure you encounter stress. Just about everyone has stress.

In the context of this book, in my humble opinion, it is how you handle this long-term stress at work that determines whether or not you will be an effective employee, manager, or business owner.

Most of us full-time employees spend most of our waking days at work. We interact with our coworkers on a continual basis. If you really think about it, coworkers are really our "work family." We rarely get to choose who is in this family.

But think about it. We are brought together with a bunch of strangers from different walks of life to share time together for the benefit of another entity to make it money. Isn't that what it boils down to?

Here, we have our interactions, conflicts, good times, and bad times. One thing we can attest to, though, is that when there is stress in the workplace for whatever reason, everybody suffers. Stress in the work environment can be due to the overall culture of the company, but even just one employee can stress out the work atmosphere.

It is my expectation that by the time you are finished reading this book, you will have a better understanding of what causes you stress at work and what prevents you from relaxing when need be. I also want you to gain a better understanding of what is actually happening to you physically, mentally, chemically, and behaviorally when you are stressed and when you are relaxed and tools you can utilize to help you relax in order to perform your best.

I also want to touch upon why it is important to know how to relax at work because the benefits are numerous. They can and will carry over into your home life as well.

In addition, I want to instruct you on ways to destress your workspace. Whether your workspace is open; a six-by-six cubicle; or a large, fancy office, there are numerous ways you can "zen" your workspace that will encourage you be more relaxed. I want you to graciously deal with the unavoidable stressors that take place during you workday. I want you to "work in zen."

Finally, and most importantly, I want you to take care of yourself. You should be the most important person in your life, even if you don't feel that way now. How can you do well at work if you are paralyzed with stress, anxiety, anger, and uncertainty? You can't. How can you effectively take care of others if you aren't your best? Let me tell you—it can be really difficult to put yourself first, especially when you have out-of-work stressors and commitments as well. I'll give you some suggestions to follow in order to get you to refocus your calm, thereby allowing you to do excellent work.

Disclaimer: Please know that I totally understand that stress is a very serious issue in and out of the workplace. One way to deal with stress (which will be talked about later) is to use humor. At times, I'll use humor in this book to help make my points, when appropriate.

But first, let me tell you my story.

I was born in Fort Wayne, Indiana into a middle-income family on St Patrick's Day—March 17.

From an early age, I knew I wanted to be a doctor. In about third grade, my mom had a meeting with my teacher, who told my mom that I was doing very well in school but that she saw children like me grow up and not do much with their life because they did not have a sense of direction. So my mom sat me down and asked what I wanted to be when I grew up. I replied that I wanted to be a doctor. At that time, I resolved in my mind that what it meant to be a doctor was that you had to want to help sick people get better and you had to be smart. That was it. My mind was made up.

I then went through elementary and middle school and did well. I played the flute and oboe in various band activities through high school. I worked when I was in high school and held three jobs during my senior year. I was able to pay for my first year of college with the money I had saved from working. I then attended college at Purdue University in West Lafayette, Indiana. While in college, I joined an amazing sorority, Zeta Phi Beta Sorority, Inc., This is where I met lifelong friends. I also worked in our student union during college to help me meet my college expenses. I had fun and did well in my classes, and while experiencing some adversity, I managed to keep my dream of being a doctor alive. After I graduated college, I attended graduate school at Indiana University in Indianapolis, Indiana, where I was preparing myself to attend medical school while I earned my Master's degree in Medical Science.

With unfaltering love and support from my family and my own tenacity, I eventually got into medical school. I took a chance and went to medical school at Rowan University College of Osteopathic Medicine in Southern New Jersey. I didn't know one person in New Jersey when I initially moved there. It was just me and my now dearly departed dog Peechez. This was a great experience in so many ways.

If you don't personally know any doctors, I'll explain that a medical school education typically lasts four years. The first two years are dedicated to classroom work, and the last two years are clinical experiences. In these clinical settings, the student can start to appreciate the rigors of a practicing physician. Although learning all you can during your rotations can definitely produce stress, the full responsibility of the patients' outcome isn't really yours. I mean, you are a student. Anyhow, I graduated medical school and became a doctor!

I chose family medicine as my specialty because I wanted to treat different patient populations. I understood that a family practice physician has to learn and know a little bit about a lot of different areas of medicine and when it's appropriate to treat or refer to a specialist as compared to a specialist, who has to know a lot about a specific area of medicine.

In residency, there were certainly some stressful times. A few times, I had to break down and go off to shed a couple of tears and then return to work. Again, I gained more insight into what an autonomously practicing attending would endure. (An "attending physician, for lack of better word is the lead physician for the patient. She is the doctor responsible for the patient's medical care until discharge home or transfer to another facility.)

In medical school, they didn't really teach us how to handle stress, or if they did, I was too stressed to understand how to manage it productively. However, one thing I did do was take it upon myself to get regular massages and pedicures. This was so relaxing for me. It provided an escape and release from my stress. It was also a time for recharging physically and mentally. I finally finished my residency and was done.

I was recruited out of residency to a small West Texas town called Pecos. After arriving, I had the realization that I was the attending physician, and the responsibility of patient welfare was on me. I did well, and more responsibility was placed on me. I started building up my patient load.

In my daily grind, I appeared happy and pleasant on the outside, and for the most part, I am this person.

But I had a secret. As my workload was increasing, my coping skills were decreasing. I was stressed the @%&* out. I felt overwhelmed, tired, sleepy, unorganized, anxious, and angry. My desk had papers and charts everywhere and I was behind on charting, answering calls, and checking labs. I would have dizzy spells and headaches, something was always hurting somewhere, and I was overweight. There would be many times I would go to the restroom and cry. I mean really cry. No one would know because I would come back out my "happy self."

Let me take a quick detour right now and tell you another secret. I really like to consider myself a non-judgmental person, and I really believe to each his own. However, I did hold consternation against people who would intentionally take their lives. I felt anger as well as sympathy for them, but I would think to myself, "What could be so bad that they would want to take their lives? How could they do that?" I thought these people were weak and selfish. I would think, "Who are you to determine when your life should end? How arrogant of you." Keep this in mind.

So now I am back at work feeling stressed, overwhelmed, and tired, and I had a *big* wake-up call. It was like cold water was splashed on my face. I was sitting at my desk one day with a look in my eyes. My medical assistant sat down on the opposite side of my desk and saw me looking sad. She caringly asked, "Dr. Gorman, is there anything I can do to help you?" I looked at her and replied, "There is nothing anyone can do to help me." She then replied how concerned she was to hear me say this, because this is what people who want to kill themselves say. I was kind of taken aback! I thought for a brief moment and replied that I could actually see why a person would just want to be done with it all. It was just too much. I just couldn't believe I was thinking this way! Wow!

My mom is alive and still encourages me to this day. I have my sisters who love me. I have my fiancé who is a support. I have my work family who is always there as well. And not *one* of them really knew what it was like for me. I really didn't feel like I could talk to anyone who would truly understand. The only one who would close to understanding would have been another doctor, but I didn't want to bother them. I also didn't want the stigma of a doctor seeking help. So yes, for that brief moment, I could see how someone could contemplate suicide. This was really a low point for me. I really felt ashamed and embarrassed.

I did have faith to realize that through the lowness must come the assent. I wanted to become a more inwardly positive and thoughtful person. I knew the major reason why I journeyed into this dark space was multifactorial, but the whole foundation was that I was stressed and unable to relax. I didn't manage my stress well. I was snapping at people for no reason, like my mom, who only offered love and support. That was not right of me. Again, how ashamed I was.

After this moment, three things happened to me. One is that I decided I never wanted to feel this way again. I was tired of being stressed out and anxious about everything all the time. Even when I was not at work, I was thinking about being at work, that I had missed something, or that I was about to be called even when I wasn't on call! It was a mess. No way to live.

Secondly, I had just returned from a conference in Atlanta where I had been given the opportunity to change the course of my life starting with my mindset and get out in the world and fulfill my dreams, and I took it. I figured out through this extraordinary shift in my mindset that if I want something different, I must do something different.

Thirdly, I decided that in addition to being a physician, one of my purposes in life is to help other stressed individuals in the work environment be made aware that not being able to get a hold on chronic stress is literally killing them. I don't want other people to get in and stay in that dark place that I visited.

I had to get out there spreading knowledge that stress doesn't have to make you sick or kill you.

I am taking the time to write this book to share with the world my story to let those out there know they are not alone when it comes to not being able to handle stress well. Stress that occurs in the work place is a major cause of mental and physical issues. People call in sick to work. People are unproductive. People are overwhelmed, uncertain, sad, and frustrated at work. It doesn't always have to be like this.

I want people to be able to calm their minds and relax their bodies, specifically in the work setting, because many of our waking hours are spent in the work setting. And as we all have stress in our lives, it should not get the best of us. I don't want anyone to get into that dark place that I was in without getting help to get out. I want to contribute to preventing someone from having a heart attack or a stroke any chronic condition whose baseline malfunction is not being able to handle their stress.

I hope that reading this book will give you the understanding, knowledge, and tools to make mindful decisions on how you personally choose to decrease your perceived stress in the work setting and emerge a healthy, productive, and fulfilled person.

Relax Well.

Chapter 1

EVALUATING THE CAUSE OF YOUR STRESS AT WORK

Before we combat your stress, you need to evaluate why you perceive you have stress at work. Right?

Workload and responsibilities placed on you at work can cause so much stress. You want to do a good job, but just the thought of what you need to accomplish can make you feel overwhelmed.

On the other hand, there are people out there who feel better if they are extra busy, and when there is down time, they feel very anxious because they want something to do. This can cause them stress.

Here are some things that are known to cause stress in the work environment.

Unrealistic Deadlines

What's more stressful than having a task placed before you and then having it due yesterday? Having unrealistic deadlines is a setup for having extra stress on so many fronts. As you take the task on, you may have to work later, which is stressful. You may lose sleep trying to get it done, which decreases your capacity to handle stress. Finally, it may take calling others in to help or finding additional resources to get it done, which is stressful. Wow.

Unrealistic Expectations

Are you being asked to do something right now that you haven't been trained to do? This can cause unnecessary stress.

Doing More Than What Is Expected

Joining extra committees, volunteering for activities, and offering to help a fellow co-worker can make things extra stressful, especially if you haven't completed your own work yet. Overextending yourself can cause a lot of stress.

Idleness

You may be one of those people who is super organized and thrives when there is work to be done. You finish it, and then there is nothing left to do. This can make you feel very stressed just sitting there waiting for the next thing to come across your path.

Work Benefits

If your income isn't meeting your living needs, this can place added pressures and stress on you, especially if you are living paycheck to paycheck and can't even think about missing a day's work. Sick days or personal days may be next to none. Is it difficult getting time to take a vacation? Do you not make enough money to save? Are you juggling bills? This can add stress to you. If you are fortunate enough to have health insurance, the coverage may not be enough. The copays and deductibles can be what determine if you buy groceries this week or not. What if you do work and are unable to be insured? The stress of thinking "what if I get sick?" is unbearable, because that will mean more bills, which causes more stress, which can make you sicker. You understand this cycle? How stressful is this?

Coworkers or Boss on Your Nerves

Is there one employee who has something to say about everything all the time, and it's usually negative? Do you deal with sarcasm, pettiness, or poor work performance that impacts your ability to do your work? Do coworkers try and pass off their responsibilities on to you? Or try and act like your boss when they are not? Do you experience stress just in anticipating having an interaction with a particular coworker? Does your coworker do nothing but complain? What about coworkers who try and kiss up to the boss? Do your coworkers gossip about others or even you? These things can all be very stressful.

Poor Management or Leadership

Not having clear direction or instruction by the "higher ups" can lead to stress. Is your boss always looking for a fight? Maybe your boss shoots down any idea that you offer. Is there always a reason not to consider your point of view? Do you not feel valued? Is your boss unreasonable? Is there no give?

On the other hand, is your boss ambiguous on what is expected of you? Is she unable to make a decision on anything? Does she change her mind when challenged on an action?

Do you have more than one person you must report to? This can be confusing. Are you being micromanaged? Does your boss instruct you to do something and then hover at every point of the process? Is your boss always grumpy? Is she miserable at work and projecting that onto you?

Poor Communication

Isn't it frustrating when there is poor communication? Do you find out about a meeting after it has already started? Or ended? Are you aware of any updated policies? Did the work schedule change and you were not informed? Is there a new deadline? Is there a particular event where attendance is mandatory and this wasn't communicated to you in time? What about issues with coworkers? Isn't it a horrible feeling to know that a coworker had an event in his family and you weren't even given the opportunity to share? I know I don't like finding out things at the last minute or after it has already happened. This is stressful.

Coworkers with Bad Work Ethic

Are your coworkers there to just get a paycheck? Perhaps their attitude is bad, they complain about everything, and their work is of poor quality. Do they have others do their work for them? Do they brown nose? Do they lie? Are they cheating? Do they have co-workers clock in/out for them? Are they having inappropriate work relationships? Do they come to work late and leave early?

All of these characteristics in a coworker can make anyone with whom they interact stressed.

Being in Management

If you are a boss, are you so busy micromanaging your employees? Isn't that tiring? Is there a shortage of employees? Are there any particular employees who are disruptive to the others and thus bringing them all down? Do you have your own supervisor hovering over you imposing deadlines? Micromanaging is stressful for you, let alone your employees.

Being a Business Owner

Suppose you are fortunate enough to own your own business. You fully understand this is your "baby". It's on you. How successful you are depends on the blueprint you develop and strategies you implement. You have your vision and values that you want to make sure are carried out. This can be very exciting, energizing, *and* stressful.

Promotion/Transfer

Have you been promoted to a higher position or transferred to another department? Being placed in a new position where there is a big learning curve or more responsibility can be stressful. If you are in new surroundings with new faces, this can cause some anxiety.

Big Changes at Work

Is there new management? Are you learning a new computer system? In my work setting, we use EMRs or electronic medical records. Let me tell you, they are no joke. Remodeling can also be a source of stress.

Uncomfortable Surroundings

You may work in an office, but it really feels like a meat locker. At the other extreme, you may be sitting at your desk roasting because someone turned up the heat. Granted you can't please everyone with the temperature, but there should be a happy medium. Either temperature extreme can cause stress because you are too uncomfortable to do your work efficiently.

Is there a lot of noise or loud music? Is the music is offensive to you? Is the lighting poor or too bright? Is there excessive dust because of remodeling? Is it flaring up your allergies? Has there not been a housekeeper in days? Having a dirty environment is not conducive to productive work and can be stressful.

Poor Support System

If you run into trouble, have questions, or have cause for concern, do you feel that you have a place you can go or a person with whom you can speak who can help you resolve this? If you do not, your stress may understandably be elevated.

Even if you actually really enjoy your job, you still cannot escape stress.

Write down five things that you feel cause you stress at work.

1. _____
2. _____
3. _____
4. _____
5. _____

Things To Remember

Things To Remember

Things To Remember

Things To Remember

Things To Remember

Chapter 2

TOXIC WORK ENVIRONMENTS

What is a toxic work environment? Well, it's actually exactly what it sounds like—an environment that is poisonous, dangerous, sickly, hurtful, apathetic, adversarial, and downright negative. Have you ever walked into a place of business or had a job interview at a potential employer and as soon as you walked in, your felt something more than your upset nerves? Have you walked in and felt that something isn't right? That there is just a vibe of negativity, bad energy, or tension? Are you working in that place right now? In my opinion, work should not be a place where the dead go to gather—unless you work at a mortuary.

How you can tell if you are in a toxic work environment? Here are some clues:

You can't be yourself at work or be permitted to have some individuality.

You can't laugh, or if there is laughter, it's at the expense of someone else, and maybe that someone is you (in a bad way).

You approach your boss with a concern or suggestion and you get shut down before you even get your sentence out.

Your boss is defensive.

You are not given the opportunity to voice your opinion when asked.

There is lack of communication in your workplace.

You don't have support or resources to do your job.

There is mistreatment of workers.

There is no professionalism at the appropriate times.

You don't have a clear understanding of your job description or adequate training to perform your job.

Indecisiveness from decision makers or no one knows what's going on

There is a lack of mutual respect.

Your boss just focuses on your mistakes and does not acknowledge your successes.

There is sabotage in the workplace.

There is inconsistent application of policies and procedures.

There is a culture "punch in, punch out" without a care for quality of work.

Coworkers are gossiping about others.

This is a long list, and I'm sure there are others. But let me ask you this. Are you yourself contributing to a toxic work environment? No one wants to believe they are. But you could be. Just think about it.

I bring this subject to light because at the end of the day, if you are working in a toxic work environment, it can be very stressful in the long term. How would you be able to relax in a contaminated place? How can you be expected to perform your best if you are not in an atmosphere designed for you to succeed?

How can you handle yourself in this type of environment, or even if it's worth you trying? Only you can determine this. If you really don't have a choice, there are ways to help you better cope. You need to know when and how to destress at work.

Do you feel that your place of employment is toxic?

List five reasons why or why not.

1. _____

2. _____

3. _____

4. _____

5. _____

Things To Remember

Things To Remember

Things To Remember

Things To Remember

Chapter 3

DEALING WITH CHALLENGING COWORKERS

Do you work in a competitive environment where how much you make depends on how much you sell? Are employees sabotaging you? Are they talking behind your back?

Most of us really don't get to pick who we work with, and even if we do, they still can be a challenge to work with. The people we work with are with us at least eight hours a day or more if we work full time.

You may have the "pleasure" of working a person who always complains about literally everything—their job, their boss, their family, you, me, their dog, the weather, you name it. You could place this coworker in a room with puppies wearing detachable $100 bill collars and this coworker still wouldn't smile. These people are unfortunately just miserable, and they may or may not realize that they are this way.

If you work with someone who isn't doing their job correctly and your ability to do your job correctly is contingent on their doing their job correctly, this can increase your stress and anxiety.

There's the coworker who is into everyone's business and then shares it with others. These are the gossips.

There may be an employee who is a bully.

Is there an employee who has personal hygiene issues? Does he have body odor? Offensive breath? Does she wear too much perfume? Does she play her music too loud? Is the smell of the food they brought for lunch very offensive?

How can we deal with these challenging people and situations? Below are some tips.

Be the Person You Want to Be Around

If you are tired of your coworker complaining about everything, then you shouldn't complain yourself. If you don't like your coworker constantly talking about someone else and gossiping, then you shouldn't talk or gossip about someone else. If you don't like back stabling, then don't do it. If you prefer to be around someone who is pleasant, be pleasant. If you like working in a cohesive team, be a team player yourself. If you like working with someone who does their job professionally, you do this as well. Just like bad attitudes can spread, so can good ones. So have a great attitude and let it "infect" the whole place.

Work in Respect

When you are working alongside multiple people with different backgrounds, religious views, political views, and personalities, no two people are going to think the same or act the same. Respect of these differences is key to thriving in a work environment. Appreciating and understanding this concept while doing your job will alleviate significant conflicts and thus decrease workplace stress. Agree that people are different and keep it moving. You are all there for the benefit of the company you work for. After all, a pot of soup needs more than one ingredient to taste good.

Pick Your Battles

Don't continually complain. When you constantly complain to others about the same issue over and over, especially if it can't or won't change anything, you are contributing to a toxic work environment. When you do this, you yourself will be labeled as the complainer and the challenging coworker. This will lead to people not taking you seriously. Sometimes you have to let it go and pick your battles. It is what it is.

Talk to the Person Who Is Stressing You

Talk to the person one on one if it is a coworker or friend. If it's someone you know, she may not be too offended. Mention that it seems that she is acting different and inquire if there something going on with them. This mention may be just enough to make them realize that their behavior is troublesome. If it's an extremely personal issue and you are a friend, this approach may be taken with gratitude, but no matter how it comes out, it will be hurtful.

If you don't know the person too well, you will likely need to get human resources involved. Go speak to them and see if there are any policies for handling the situation. Maybe you can look in your employee handbook, make a copy, and anonymously place it on your coworker's desk. If there is a conflict that can't be hashed out on the personal level, human resources can be an arbitrator.

Keep in mind that just the same way you wouldn't appreciate someone talking about you, it's only respectful not to talk about someone else, even if you don't get along. And if someone comes to talk to you, please keep an open mind because it may be a valid issue—something you yourself didn't realize.

Avoid the Person

Now I'm not talking about going into hiding or ducking for cover if you see them walking towards you, but if you have the occasion to be in contact with a coworker who is challenging for you, politely keep it moving. Walk away or change the subject. If they are in your face talking about the issue, just mention that you don't have time to talk about it or now isn't a good time to talk.

Report Sexual Harassment and Bullying

Bullying and harassment are other unacceptable behaviors at work, or anywhere else, for that matter, and should not be tolerated in any form. For the recipient, it is obviously stressful because they are on the receiving end. No one likes to be talked about in a negative manner, isolated, made fun of, humiliated, or made to feel less than. Even being looked at inappropriately can be considered bullying or harassment. It goes further than this. Bullying doesn't have to be physical. It can be mental. If someone is made to feel bad because they did or did not do something, this is considered bullying. If someone is manipulated into doing something they don't want to do, this is also considered bullying. If a person is made to feel threatened in any manner, this is bullying. If a person is being put in the spotlight of intimidation or jokes because of the color of their skin, religious background, body habits, or disability, this is harassment. The stress of the recipient, I'm sure, is at the highest level.

If you are dealing with more grave work issues like bullying or sexual harassment, there are definitely a few things you can do, because you do have the right to work in a non-hostile environment.

Something as simple as a coworker putting her hand on your shoulder and giving you a "neck massage" without you asking for it can be considered sexual harassment.

Other examples of sexual harassment are:

- Making sexually suggestive statements
- Showing a coworker inappropriate sexual pictures or pornographic websites
- Sexual innuendo (talking about something sexual without overtly saying it)
- Staring at a person sexually
- Asking personal, sexually oriented questions
- Making jokes about sexuality, sexual orientation, or sexual practices
- Overt gestures like placing your hand on someone's face, bottom, or chest.
- Holding someone's hand, brushing against someone, or standing very close to a person and they are noticeably uncomfortable
- Commenting on how a person looks sexually (for example saying "That's a nice shirt" vs. saying "I like how that shirt fits your chest")
- Sending unwanted sexually charged emails, letters, or phone messages

No one wants to feel like they are not valued as an person let alone at work as an employee. Being bullied, no matter where the setting, is serious issue. We have all known someone or even been the person who has been bullied, and it's not enjoyable. It is demoralizing, humiliating, and frankly unnecessary. Undoubtedly, it causes stress. Here are a few examples of what is considered bullying in the workplace:

- Exclusion from activities
- Being talked about
- Being ignored
- Making one person the end of a practical joke
- Constant criticism of a person
- Yelling at someone in front of others or in private
- Spreading rumors about a person
- Calling someone names (derogatory or suggestive)
- Pushing or even nudging someone
- Withholding information from someone that you know is needed for them to do their job
- Making a person believe that they will be liked if they do a particular thing

Look in your employee handbook and see if there are any policies for dealing with these serious issues. It should tell you what you need to do to proceed further. When you contact and file a complaint with human resources, they are obligated to investigate.

You need to document what is going on. This includes what happened, the date and time, and if someone else was there to witnesses it. Take note if your employer has video in the workplace. Do what you have to do to document it. Keep this documentation at home in safe place.

Seek counsel from a professional (e.g. doctor, therapist, pastor). This is a trusted professional, so you can speak freely, and they can also document what has been told to them.

You may have to seek legal counsel to see your options to proceed.

Seek counsel from a trusted family member or friend. They can be that listening ear or shoulder on which to cry.

Plan Your Exit Strategy

Sometimes you have to realize that enough is enough. Have you done all you can do, and talked to everyone you can? I am not advocating walking off the job. Unless you are in imminent physical danger, I don't really believe in burning bridges if you can help it. But you need to ask yourself if can you just continue to float, tread water, see the shark and try to fight it, or swim to shore and go look for another beach. In other words, do you just try and get by where you are, or do you say, "I've had enough" and go look for someplace else?

One final thought. Now that I have said all of this, if in the future someone approaches you and wants to talk to you, you have to "eat it". Please keep an open mind. Listen to what is being said and see if there is any validity to what this person is saying. Try not to be defensive. Even if you don't agree, have the dignity to have a discussion. Because I'm sure it's taking a lot of courage to even approach you in the first place. Whether it's a friend or a non-friend, just be calm, take a deep breath, and listen.

In summary, you can deal with challenging coworkers by:

1. Being the person you want to be around
2. Working in respect
3. Picking your battles
4. Talking to the person
5. Avoiding the person
6. Reporting sexual harassment and bullying

List five things that you find challenging in a coworker:

1. _____
2. _____
3. _____
4. _____
5. _____

For each challenge written above, how do you propose you will resolve this challenge?

1. _____
2. _____
3. _____
4. _____
5. _____

Things To Remember

Things To Remember

Things To Remember

Things To Remember

Chapter 4

STRESS CAN AFFECT YOU PHYSICALLY, CHEMICALLY, HORMONALLY, MENTALLY, EMOTIONALLY, AND BEHAVIORALLY

When you are acutely stressed, your sympathetic nervous system is activated. This is your "fight or flight" nervous system. It is activated in times of stress or perceived threat. The parasympathetic nervous system, on the other hand, is the "rest and digest" part of the nervous system. This is activated when you are relaxing, eating, and using the restroom.

Did you know that stress affects you in many different ways? Some of these ways are ways listed below.

Physical

Physical stress causes tension in your muscles. You may feel pain. You feel uptight because you are always tensing your muscles. You might not even know you are doing it. Here, I have shown you a few of the muscles that are affected when you are stressed.

There is a large back muscle called the trapezius, which inserts at the base of your head (the occiput), travels down the middle of your back (the thoracic spine), and fans out to the shoulder blades (the scapulae). Here, we have illustrated the top part of that muscle. We also have the splenius capitus and semispinalis capitus, which attach to back of head. They support your head and neck and move them. The levator scapuli is a muscle that helps to lift up the shoulder blade (scapula).

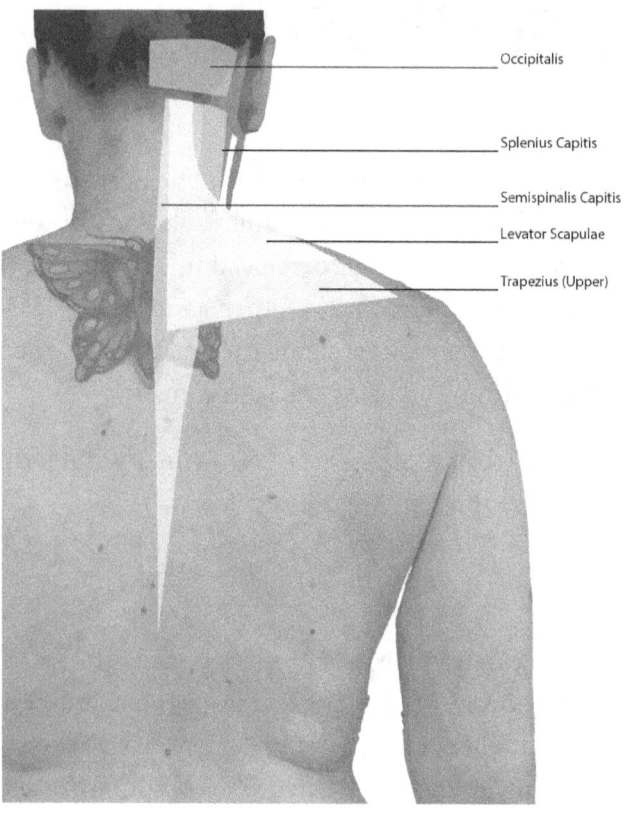

There are muscles in your face, head, and front neck that can also become tensed when you are stressed.

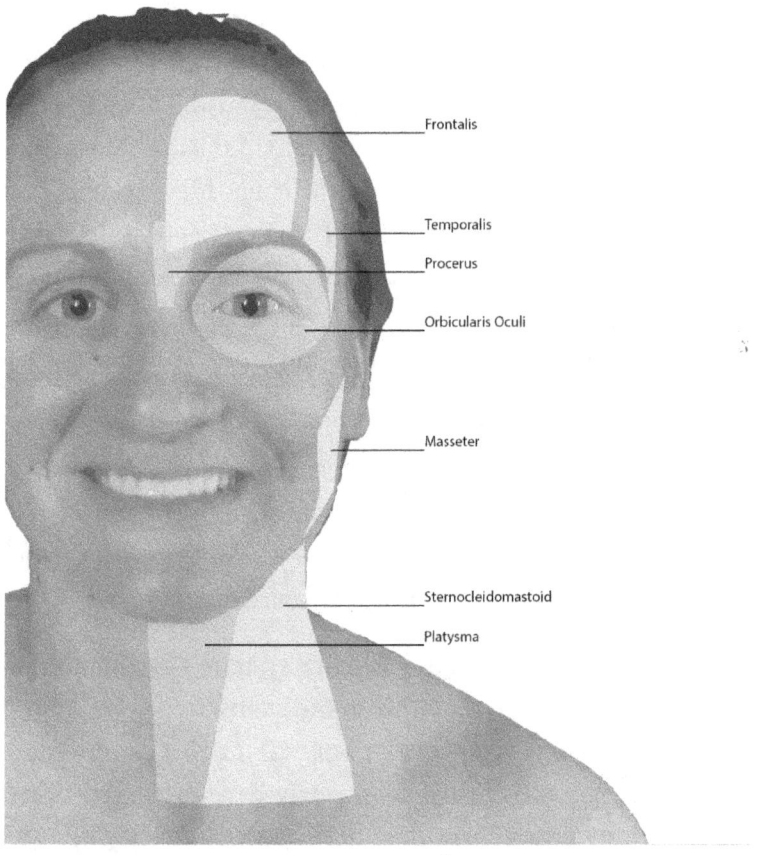

The frontalis muscle helps you to wrinkle your forehead and raises the eyebrows, for example, when you frown. The temporalis muscle is on the side of the head and moves the jaw and helps with chewing. The procerus muscle is located on the base of the forehead and the top of nasal bone. It helps you to frown. The orbicularis oculus is a muscle that surrounds your eye. This muscle is responsible for closing your eye lid. The masseter is one of the muscles you use when you chew. This muscle is clenched when you are stressed. The sternocleidomastoid helps to turn your head and flex the neck. Finally, there is the platysma. This is a large broad muscle that attaches the lower jaw (mandible) and the collar bone (clavicle). It covers the sternocleidomastoid. The playstisma pulls down the lower lip and side of mouth and jaw. It's also a muscle of facial expression. Finally, just for extra knowledge, this muscle is a contributor to the "double chin."

Yes, *all* of these muscles can become tensed or strained and cause discomfort. That's how tension headaches happen. This is why you have more neck pain when you are stressed. You can also have jaw pain because you are clenching your jaw without even realizing it. Make sense now?

Concerning your gastrointestinal system, your "guts" may be in an uproar. Even though you can't consciously and physically control how your digestive system works, it can and does physically respond to stress. You may have increased heartburn or indigestion. You may have more loose stools, especially when anxious about something such as preparing to give a speech.. Constipation may also be an issue.

Mental/Emotional

Mental manifestations of stress include anxiety, panic attacks, depression, anger, and fear. These are not productive. The mental anguish of stress is certainly real. Constantly thinking of what needs to be done is stressful. Adding a deadline to something makes it all the worse. Oh yes, I totally understand that when you are at work, you must meet deadlines. Having this constant worry can set you up for anxiety or having panic attacks. The bare thought of something imminent or in the future may make your chest tighten, your breathing rate increase, your skin crawl, or your stomach nauseous. Basically, when you think of something, it can freak you out. This is a panic or anxiety attack. **Anxiety** is an overall sense of panic from the inside out. It is an inner uneasiness or constant worry about something that is a perceived theat. It can be really devastating and paralyzing for some people. Anticipating having to do something (give a speech is a big one) or go somewhere (a crowded place) can produce anxiety in people. It is definitely a source of stress, and the same hormones responsible for the stress response are released when one feels anxious. Fear is a feeling of being threatened, which can also lead to anxiety. Fear can be of both the known and the unknown.

Another manifestation of uncontrolled stress is **depression**. Depression is a medical condition diagnosed by meeting certain criteria. Most people at some point in their lives will have a touch of depression, but do you get to a point where you can't cope with life or care for yourself? If you feel that, you may be depressed more than what is normal for you. If this is the case, I would recommend being properly examined and counseled.

Anger is an emotion that can manifest itself as frustration. Why are you angry? Is it because you are disappointed? Do you feel a lack of control over a situation? Do you feel bad that you are unable to control this emotion?

Fear is an emotion at the center of stress. When you don't know when something is going to happen, you can feel stressed about it. When you do know about something that is going to happen and you are in anticipation of the known, this can cause stress. Anytime you feel threatened, this brings up anxiety and thus stress.

Chemical/Hormonal

Chemically, being stressed causes the release of "stress hormones" in your body. Let's back up first. What are hormones? Hormones are chemical messengers secreted by glands. Well, what are glands? Glands are structures in the body that secrete substances. We have exocrine glands and endocrine glands. An exocrine gland secretes substances into a duct, like your salivary or spit gland, and have a proximal (close to) effect. An endocrine gland secretes hormones into the blood stream to affect other areas in the body. The glands responsible for making these "stress hormones" are called the adrenal glands.

The adrenal glands are two little structures that sit on the top of your kidneys. In times of stress, these glands secrete hormones.

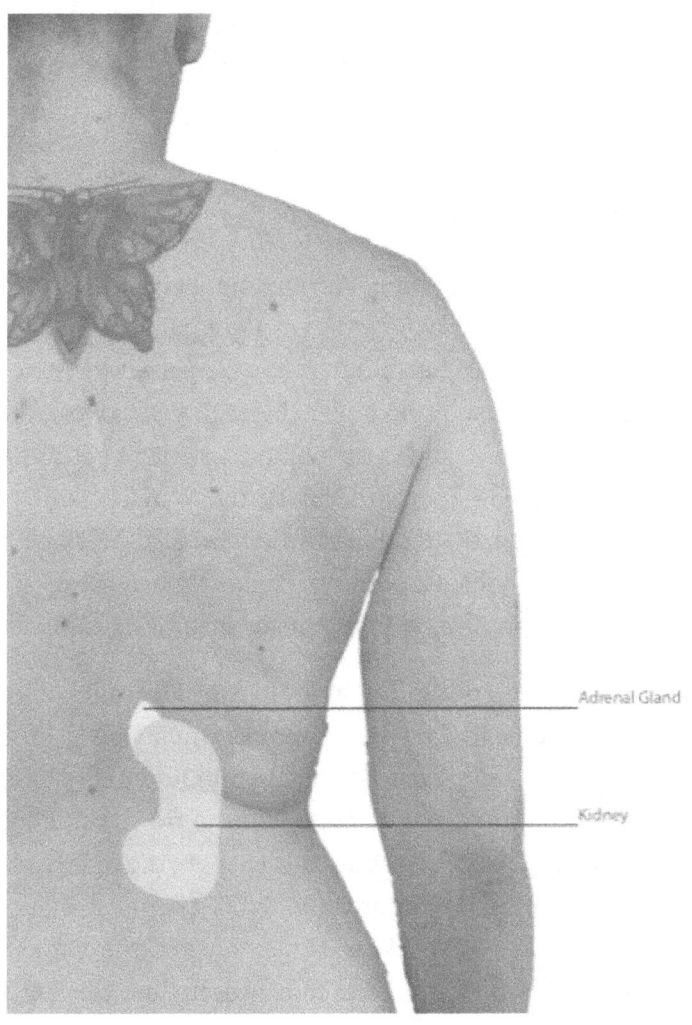

At this point, I should also mention neurotransmitters before I continue. Don't worry, I will make it simple for you to understand. To put it simply, nerves (neurons) communicate with one another via neurotransmitters. Neurotransmitters are types of hormones that, once released from one nerve, travel to a nearby nerve so that the recipient nerve can be activated and perform its function—either an emotional response, physical movement, or bodily function.

The stress hormones are:

Adrenalin (epinephrine): Adrenaline helps to stimulate the sympathetic nervous system. Remember that fight or flight mechanism? When adrenalin is present, it increases heart rate, opens up the bronchioles (breathing passages), increases blood pressure, and dilates blood vessels to get more blood flow to the body parts that need them and constricts blood flow to the parts that don't. Adrenalin also helps with carbohydrate metabolism, meaning it helps to increase blood sugar so that the muscles can use that sugar for energy.

Noradrenaline (norepinephrine): Noradrenalin is a "cousin" to epinephrine, but its scope of function is a little more limited. It is mainly used to obtain and maintain blood pressure. It is also a neurotransmitter. (Just a quick aside for you nerds who are actually reading this chapter, the difference between adrenalin and noradrenalin is its chemical makeup and where it reacts based on if there are receptors for it. Adrenalin is made from noradrenalin. Adrenaline can exert its effects mostly everywhere in the body, depending on the receptor for it. It is released mostly in times of stress. Noradrenaline has restricted activity based on receptor recognition and is actually responsible for keeping the blood pressure up. It is actually released continuously in the body.)

Cortisol: Cortisol is a steroid hormone that is responsible for mobilizing blood sugar stores so that sugar can be used for energy. It also breaks down fat stores into fatty acids. In addition, it is responsible for breaking down stored protein into its components called amino acids to help repair damaged cells or make enzymes for chemical reactions in your body to occur. Cortisol increases blood pressure so that blood carrying the nutrients and glucose can arrive to wherever it's going quicker.

Cortisol also suppresses the body's immune and inflammation response.

Thinking this though, cortisol increases the amounts of amino acids, blood sugar, and fatty acids in the blood and decreases inflammation and the immune response in times of stress.

Can you see where having continually elevated blood cortisol is driving you?

Glucagon: Glucagon is a hormone made in an organ called the pancreas. You may have heard of a hormone called insulin. As insulin's job is to decrease blood sugar, glucagon's job is to raise blood sugar. It is activated when your blood sugar level is too low. Glucagon is also released when you eat a protein-rich meal to help the amino acids that are formed by breaking down protein when you digest it make more glucose. It is secreted in times of stress—when adrenalin is released—again, so your body can use that sugar for energy.

Growth Hormone: Growth hormone is made in the brain. Its function in children is to literally help them grow their bodies. In adults, it helps to keep those body structures that have grown normal. In both children and adults, it helps control body metabolism. Growth hormone is not released continually in the body, but in bursts. Its levels are increased when blood sugar is low and during exercise, sleep, and—you got it—stress. Growth hormone acts to increase blood sugar and fatty acids to use for times of stress.

In summary, these hormones work to do a bunch of things. When your body is prepared to move quickly or perceives danger or stress, they kick in. Your heart rate and blood pressure increase to move blood quicker to the muscles and organs that need it. Sugar is made or released quickly to supply those running muscles with energy to get out of there. Your breathing rate increases. This is great when you need to get something done quickly. Then, the hormones return to a normal level.

BUT…

When your body is in a chronically stressed state, those hormones are still elevated. Those stress hormones also affect other hormones in your body that were just sitting there minding their own business. Boy oh boy does having uncontrolled stress play a huge role in why we have so many health issues. Chronic uncontrolled stress contributes to:

- High blood pressure or hypertension
- Insulin resistance/diabetes
- Polycystic ovarian syndrome
- Obesity
- Belly fat
- Chronic headaches/migraines
- Hair loss
- Depression
- Anxiety
- Frequent colds
- Acid reflux disease
- Chronic fatigue
- Irritable bowel syndrome
- Cardiovascular disease (heart attack/stoke)

- Insomnia
- Low sex drive
- Erectile dysfunction
- Irregular periods
- Pre-menstrual syndrome
- Body aches
- Muscle aches
- Joint pain
- Weakened immune system
- Increased risk of infection
- Rashes
- Weight gain

Are you or anyone you know affected with these conditions? If so, you might need to work to get your stress levels under control.

Behavioral

Behaviorally, stress can cause you to develop non-beneficial habits such as smoking, drinking, overeating, undereating, illegal drug use, and overutilizing prescription drugs. All of these self-destructive habits set you up for complicated health issues. Smoking damages your lung tissue, which can lead to chronic bronchitis, chronic obstructive pulmonary disorder, emphysema, and lung cancer.

Drinking alcohol can damage your liver, brain, pancreas, stomach and heart. Overstressing your liver to detoxify the chemicals can literally wear it out. Your brain and your heart can both suffer long-term effects of drinking alcohol as well.

Overeating can lead to insulin resistance and then diabetes. Overeating will set you up for heart disease, elevated cholesterol, obesity, and osteoarthritis. Undereating can lead to malnutrition, weak bones, dry skin, and hair loss.

Uncontrolled or unchanneled stress may also lead to other addictive behaviors. Addictive behaviors are behaviors or actions in which a person engages to temporarily escape an unpleasant or unwanted situation or to cope with stress but that are hard to stop. Examples of addictive behaviors are sex addiction, excessive playing of video games, or being abusive.

Why do these habits develop? These are coping mechanisms. Yet again, our amazing brain has figured out a way to help us take our mind off of stressful situations—temporarily. When you are engaging in seemingly pleasurable things, you mentally leave your stress. In the long term, however, you are self-destructing.

When you are done engaging in these harmful and non-productive habits, the stressful thing is still waiting for you. So how do you help yourself? Find a more productive way to handle your stress. This will be discussed in shortly.

Things To Remember

Things To Remember

Things To Remember

Things To Remember

Things To Remember

Chapter 5

WHAT STRESS DOES TO YOU AT WORK

Decreases Productivity

When you are tense and uptight with work, you tend not to move as much, likely due to pain. You make more mistakes because your concentration is poor. You must keep checking over what you did, which wastes time. You may not even complete your task because you may feel too overwhelmed about it. You become unmotivated to push forward. You may come to work late. You don't manage your time very well.

Worsens Your Attitude

When you are feeling stressed, it's hard to be happy and positive. Remember that attitudes are contagious. Just one person can spread their negativity to the rest of the people with whom they interact. This can spread throughout the entire workplace. You may even be angry because you are not able to deal with the stress that is befalling you, and this emotion can spread to others as well.

Fosters Isolation

Your coworkers may avoid you because you bring them down. Who wants to be around someone who is always negative, depressed, or frantic? It causes extra stress. Or even worse, you might self-isolate. You don't participate fully in your job or in your necessary interactions. It is one thing to seclude yourself because you have a deadline and need to remain free from distractions in order to get it done, but it's another to purposefully avoid others.

I totally understand that people can have good days and bad days, but you can make adjustments with your attitude so that you can function better.

Other Areas of Your Life Suffer

When you are chronically stressed, you stop taking care of yourself. When you stop taking care of yourself, you are setting yourself up for failure in so many different aspects of your life. Work is only one area that suffers. Your relationships can suffer when you bring the stresses of work home. Your spouse may feel neglected. Your children may not understand what's going on with you. Friendships may suffer. You may stop your participation in things you really enjoy doing outside of work.

Missed Workdays

As previously stated, having chronic uncontrolled stress can lead to physical illness. Your immune system is worn down due to chronic stress, which leaves your body with the inability or decreased capacity to fight off infection and disease. You shouldn't work when you are ill because you won't be able to perform at your best.

Sometimes you are not physically ill but mentally exhausted. You are "sick" of coming to work due to the stress, so you call in sick just to have a day off. I am actually a proponent of taking mental health days. You may not have a physical cold, but you are just done and don't want to deal with work life today. Now, I understand a lot of bosses may not like me to say that, but would you rather pay for an employee to sit around and do nothing or perform poorly, or have a refreshed employee ready to work, putting forth their best effort?

Name five ways you feel stress is affecting you at work:

1. _____
2. _____
3. _____
4. _____
5. _____

INTERLUDE

I can hear what you are thinking. "You have given me plenty of great information about what stress does to me, how it affects me, and how its making me sick, but *how* am I going to be helped?

Exactly how are you going to be able to help me with my stress at work, Dr. Deitrick?"

I'm glad you asked.

Keep reading.

Things To Remember

Things To Remember

Things To Remember

Things To Remember

Chapter 6

BENEFITS OF RELAXATION

Numerous benefits are seen when you are able to relax at work.

Increased Productivity

Productivity is the ability and capability to get things done. When you are more productive, you get more things done. Whenever you are calmer and more focused, you can do more and maybe even be more efficient at it.

Less Tension

This is literal and figurative. Your muscles are more relaxed, so there is less tension, less pain, more mobility, and more flexibility. Now you are poised to perform your job.

You have less mental strife when you are relaxed. The war in your mind is over, or at least decreased.

Feeling Happier

What are some of the things you feel when you are "happy"? What does being happy mean anyhow? To me, happy means being joyous, positive, optimistic, agreeable, or upbeat about something. When you feel happy, you are usually more relaxed and open to more things. Life in general just seems better.

More Energy

When you are relaxed, you have that pep in your step. It's like getting paid. When it's payday, life is just great. You get that happy walk in your stride. Even if your money already has someplace to go when you get it, you still got that pep. Now imagine if you can have that same swag with your mindset when you change the way you think about things. That's what calming your mind can do for you. It's that inner sense of peace and harmony that is uplifting, and it actually recharges your "battery" because you know it will be okay.

Better Decisions

With a clear and calm mind, you think through the pros and cons when making a decision. Decisions are not made in uneducated haste because you are not focused on being tired and wanting to rest. When you are in panic mode, you think survival. When you are in relaxation mode, you use logic when you think.

Better Understanding

When you are relaxed, you are more receptive. You obtain a better understanding all around. You are better able to understand what is expected of you at work. You also have a better understanding of what to expect from others.

Better Listening

A calm mind is a receptive mind. This is so true on so many levels. When your mind is calm, you are more open to hearing another person's point of view. You are more receptive to instructions. You hopefully can take constructive criticism with a better attitude.

To sum up most of the above, you essentially become a more effective communicator. A breakdown in communication can destroy empires, even if intensions are well laid out.

For *any* relationship, company, business, project, or mission to be successful, the top and the base must have effective communication. When your mind is stressed, tired, and disconnected, success will not happen. It just will not.

Things To Remember

Things To Remember

Things To Remember

Things To Remember

Things To Remember

Chapter 7

RELAXATION HORMONES

I talked earlier about the stress hormones and how they affect you. Now let's briefly talk about some of the relaxation or feel-good/happy hormones.

Serotonin: Serotonin is a neurotransmitter that is produced in the brain *and* the intestines. Most of it is found in the intestines. It is also found in platelets, which help our blood clot. Serotonin plays a role in our mood and anxiety. Serotonin is decreased in depression. It is elevated when we are happy and relaxed. It may also be involved in obsessive compulsive disorder (OCD). Too high or too low of levels can also be related to irritable bowel (makes sense, since it's in the intestines).

There are some natural ways that have been reported to improve serotonin levels. Exercise, being outside in sunlight, and eating foods rich in tryptophan can help. Tryptophan is an amino acid that is important in making serotonin. Taking St. John's wart can act as an anti-depressant by preventing re-uptake of serotonin and keeping it around for longer. As this is a supplement, you will definitely need to discuss this with your doctor/NP/PA, as medication interactions can occur with prescribed as well as over-the-counter drugs.

Melatonin: Melatonin is a neurotransmitter that helps to balance the sleep-awake cycle. It is made in the brain in a gland called the pineal gland. To best be able to cope with stressors of life, in my opinion, you need to be well rested from having had enough sleep the night before. People who work the night shift can have this cycle upset. People who have insomnia (the inability to have restful sleep) can also have this sleep-wake cycle disrupted. There is over-the-counter man-made melatonin. Again, speak with your doctor and see if this is something from which you may benefit if you are having difficulty sleeping.

Oxytocin: Oxytocin is a hormone that acts as a neurotransmitter. It comes from the brain. As you may or may not know, it is a player in the birthing process as well as breastfeeding. It plays a role in social interaction, trust, and bonding. It is also released in times of intimacy. When you are intimate, there is trust, relaxation, and bonding.

Oxytocin helps reduce stress and anxiety.

Dopamine: Dopamine is also a neurotransmitter. Is related to happiness and helps promote pleasure. Exercise, sunlight, and good nutrition all increase dopamine.

Endorphins: Endorphins are called endogenous morphine. What does endogenous mean? It means your body makes them. Endorphins are a group of neurotransmitters. These endorphins are released when our body perceives pain or stress to help decrease both. Endorphins interact with the same receptors in our brain that are present with addiction. They are called opiate receptors. The good thing about our own receptors and our body's natural endorphins is that it doesn't lead to the addiction that is typically thought of when we think drug addiction.

How do we raise our own natural endorphins? With pretty much everything we should be doing anyways—eating healthy, exercising, laughing, listening to nice music, meditation, being outdoors in the sun, and deep breathing.

Things To Remember

Things To Remember

Things To Remember

Things To Remember

Things To Remember

Chapter 8

HOW TO MANAGE STRESS AT WORK

Mind Your Business

Tell me how can you do your work admirably, purposefully, with integrity, and with excellence if you are worrying about how your coworker is or is not doing their job. Why would you put that stress upon yourself? Just release that worry. You can't control what someone else is doing any more than you can control the sun coming up. It's going to happen no matter what you do. Now you may be saying, "Well, I work in a group, and what one person does will dictate what I do." That is a fair concern, and I'm not downplaying that. If this is the case, my suggestion would be to approach this person with an empathic heart. Show some kindness. Ask this person what the problem is. Is he not clear on what is supposed to be done? Are they going through personal issues that are distracting them from their work life? Why is she not able to complete her part? On the other hand, if you approach this person and there is no reason for not being a team player and they just don't find this project important, then it's imperative to find someone to replace this person. No drama about it—it is what it is.

Along these same lines, you are not in elementary school, avoid being a tattle tale. You know, back in the day, there was always one student who was keeping track of everyone else when it was not even their job to and then would report to the teacher. At work, it's not your business if a person clocked in late or took an extra day off. It's stressful trying to keep track of others' whereabouts when you are not hired to do that! Mind your business and decrease that stress!

Get and Stay Organized

Get a planner. Use that planner. When you have a schedule, you can rest in the fact that you don't have to do any extra thinking. Make sure things around you are organized.

Understand Your Job, Then Do Your Job

There is a sense of calm and maybe even happiness that is fostered with clarity. If you know what is expected of you as an employee and what you expect from your employer, this will lessen your anxiety. If you are interviewing for a job, be clear of what you will be doing. As an employee, make sure you feel that you have been trained to do your job. If not, politely ask for more time to train. I would think an employer would rather take a little bit more time to make sure you understand than get rid of you, hire someone new, and then start the retraining process from scratch.

If you are a manager, it is up to you to make sure those you are charged to lead are understanding their roles. Ambiguity fosters confusion, and confusion fosters anxiety. Get it together. Get clear, and this cause of stress will melt away.

Delegate

If you are in a position to offload some of your obligations and responsibilities to others, that's exactly what you should do. Only do this, however, if you feel that you can trust the person to whom you are relinquishing your responsibility. It serves you no good to share a responsibility with another whom you are scared is not going to do the work according to your expectations. If you have to worry if it's going to be done right, this will cause you worry and then add to your stress.

Avoid Negativity

Avoid negative conversations. If you must interact with someone who is always negative or has something negative to say about everything, change the subject to something positive. Don't reply to a negative or inappropriate statement. You may literally have to walk away from them.

Go to the water cooler to get water, not to get gossip. How would you like the water cooler topic of the day to be about you? In my opinion, most people don't consider themselves to be negative.

If you have no idea what I am talking about, you may be the person who is considered the negative one. Why be negative? What purpose does it serve you or your company if there is nothing positive to contribute? Instead of spreading gossip, why not spread compliments? Instead of always being the naysayer, unless it is a truly valid point, why not just be quiet?

Laugh a Lot

Why do "they" say laughter is the best medicine? There may be some truth to that. When you are in the midst of a good laugh, your brain releases endorphins—your body's "feel good hormones." Laughing also stimulates your immune system, which can mean you are more apt to fight off disease. Laughing can also decrease pain temporarily.

Laughing improves your mood. When there is a common reason to laugh with coworkers, it will definitely lighten up the atmosphere. It will improve coworker bonding.

Laughing improves communication because when you are laughing or just had a good laugh, you are typically in good spirits. When you are in good spirits, you are more approachable and more apt to listening.

Laughing can decrease your anxiety. There's a release when you are laughing. Exhaling when laughing and contracting and relaxing abdominal muscles is a tension buster.

Laughing can actually improve your productivity and creativity by putting you in a better mood, so now your mind is more open and ideas can flow. This will increase your productivity. Now on the other hand, unless your profession is a comedian, you can't be sitting around all day telling jokes and laughing it up, as this is nonproductive. But you understand my point.

Laughing can definitely deescalate a conflict (or escalate it, depending on the timing). If you find yourself not seeing eye to eye with your boss or coworker, you may be able to slide in a remark or witty comment that can lighten the mood. But please, if you don't think it would help, don't do it, as this may make it worse.

One final thought—it's never appropriate to laugh if it causes another person harm.

Try laughing at yourself too!

Let It Go

I'm telling you, when you come to the realization that "it is what it is," it is so freeing. A weight is lifted off. Let go of the illusion of being able to control something you cannot. Just how you can't control when a dog barks at a stranger, you can't control if someone will get upset at you for even saying hi. You really can't control what another person thinks about you. You can't control what another person says about you. There's really only one person you can control, and this person is—wait for it—you.

Just let all the crap go. If it's not directly and physically causing you harm, let it go. You can train your mind to deal with negative thoughts. Really just release it. Let it go.

Admit Your Mistakes, Apologize, and Keep It Moving

You are human. I am human. Okay, now that this is established, understand that mistakes will be made, yes, even at work. So, when you make a mistake, are you the one to quickly admit it and try to correct it, or do you spend all your much-needed time trying to hide it or manipulate it in some way to make it appear that you didn't make a mistake? Isn't the latter exhausting and mentally draining? It's hard to remember a lie, so don't do it. Every action has a consequence. If you have to eat the mistake, just do it. It is such a liberation of your mind to release error and guilt. I wish I could say if you admit a mistake, the consequence will be the equivalent to eating apple pie on a beach, but this may not be the case. But having said that, when you walk in the truth, it is calming. Try it. Remember, it is what it is.

Dress Cute and Comfy

You can definitely look cute in work clothes. You don't have to feel like you are a stuffed sausage to do it either. When you are dressed in comfortable clothing, you are relaxed. You can breathe. If business attire is your work wear, be comfy in it. If you are a nurse, wear your cute scrubs. Whatever uniform you are required to wear, make sure it's the right size. You should be able to more around.

Wear comfortable shoes to work. What is worse than working at a job where you can barely move or breathe because your clothes are malfunctioning. You have nothing to prove to others by the way you dress unless you are a designer.

Keep a sweater or light jacket available for temperature changes. Being too hot or too cold at work can make you more strained and less focused.

One more thing. No matter where you work, I would recommend you having an extra change of clothes as well as toiletry products at your work or at least in your car that you can easily get to in case there is an emergency. I don't know how I inherited the "spill food on shirt" gene. But every time I eat something, no matter how careful I try to be, I spill something on my top! It's quite an amazing talent. Knowing I have something near me that I can change into when necessary decreases my stress. Come to think of it, I should come out with a line of adult bibs. I know I can't be the only one who would benefit.

Take Potty Breaks

Really. What's worse than having a full bladder or the relentless urge to go number two when you are under pressure to get work done? You can't think. You can't concentrate. You feel anxious. You may even have pain. Just go to the restroom, please. It's a literal and figurative release. Don't forget to use your spray afterwards, or you will cause stress for the person who comes behind you!

Shout It Out

Haven't you ever wanted so badly to say to someone exactly what you are thinking or how you feel about them personally? What about a particular situation at work or a new work policy that has been implemented that you don't agree with? You keep talking to the bosses about a particular issue, and they are just not listening to you. You want speak or *shout* something because it's just boiling inside of you, and you are about to explode, but you know if you say it, you will get fired or lose a relationship. Well, I'm here to tell you that you *can* do all of this. You can say *exactly* what you want to say, how you want to say it. But there's only one condition.

You have to do it in your car. With the windows rolled up. Tightly. I know this may sound different, but I'm telling you, it's a release. Immediate release. It is really great. I have done it, and I immediately felt better and actually found myself laughing at the end. Please just try it.

If you are concerned someone will see you, you can hold your phone up to your ear like you are talking to someone.

Just try it once!

Say No

This is a powerful word. If you are a very agreeable person, this may be difficult for you to do. But practice. If you want to say it in a nicer way, you can say, "I am not able to at this time due to other obligations" or "Now is not a good time for me to do this." It's such a release of that stress to say no. It is finite.

Use Proper Body Mechanics

Having your workspace set up such that it causes you the least amount of muscle tension is of great benefit. Is your back supported? You can put something in your chair that supports your back muscles. You can also use a foot support where your feet are elevated. This decreases lower back muscle tension. Is your computer screen in an optimal location where your neck is not in an awkward position? Also remember that staring at a screen too long can cause eye strain and headaches.

Things To Remember

Things To Remember

Things To Remember

Things To Remember

Things To Remember

Chapter 9

MINDFUL RELAXATION AT WORK

What does mindful mean? It means making a conscious decision to pay attention or to engage. So, when I say mindful, I want you to be fully engaged in these relaxation techniques so that you can really gain some benefit.

Engage All Your Senses

Hear

Listen to music that is calming and relaxing or pleasant and familiar. Purchase a commercial-free app that plays music or specifically has medication music. Listening to music with which you are familiar will place you in a good mood, possibly bring back fond memories, and lighten your worries. Listening to calm music can no doubt put you in the right mind frame of relaxation.

Touch

Use your sense of touch to dissipate nervous energy. Have you ever seen a Zen sand garden? Using the rake by making curves or swirlies on the inside of the garden creates the feeling of relaxation. Using a stress ball not only strengthens your hand and lower arm muscles, but it can help release tension by relaxing those intentionally tightened muscles. It's an instant relief. There are other toys that you can put on your desk that are designed to relieve stress.

Taste

There are plenty of healthy foods and snacks that can help decrease stress. There are healthier alternatives than the traditional chips and candies, which although are delicious, are not the best for overall health in the long term. Common snacks you can have at work that are known to fight stress include:

- Fruits: bananas, cherries, blueberries, oranges, lemon, grapefruit, kiwi, strawberries, and avocadoes. Uh, are you thinking smoothie? I am!

- Vegetables: broccoli, asparagus, spinach, sweet potatoes, seaweed

- Nuts/Seeds/Beans: almonds, walnuts, pistachios, beans

- Meats: turkey, beef, salmon, shrimp

- Other: dark chocolate, oatmeal, Greek yogurt, whole grains

- Drinks: decaffeinated teas (chamomile), warm milk, lemon tea, water

These items have zinc, B vitamins, and magnesium, which are good to have on board when your body is stressed.

Make sure you are mindfully snacking. Be aware that you are eating. Enjoy the flavors. If you are diabetic, you may want to combine the fruits with something richer in protein so that your sugars don't rise to quickly.

As you can see, there are a lot of choices, so go ahead and make that salad or smoothie for lunch! Just remember one thing. Save me some!

Smell

What can I tell you? Using your sense of smell is the best. When I smell this old-school lotion (brand name excluded, cherry almond flavor), it brings me back to childhood. It's one of my favorite scents. It just makes me feel so good and happy to smell it. That's what's so great about your sense of smell. There are so many scents that calm you down. Lavender is known to relax your mood. Among others are rose, lilac bergamot, and chamomile. One scent that you love may not be the best for another. Just try some new things. Even smelling certain foods or drinks can give you a calm feeling.

I suggest using an essential oil diffuser if you have your own office. Depending on what kind of a day I am having, I use more drops. If it's an over-the-top day, I find myself turning the bottle upside down. If you are in a smaller area or have a shared workspace, you want to use a scent that doesn't travel too far. I would suggest using a personal spray mister or roll-on scent that you can use randomly to give your senses a pick me up—or rather a calm me down! If misters and roll-on scents are not your thing, I will suggest you hang a small scent diffuser close enough to you.

If you are involved in a loving, happy, and kindhearted relationship, what better fun way to have that person "near you" than to spray their favorite scent on an index card and place in a plastic Ziploc bag or the like before you go to work. When you are at work and you want a more tangible way to remember that special person and bring a smile to your face, just smell it. It will remind you of all the good things about that special person, thus calming you down.

Candles are a great way to scent up a space, but don't even think about using one at work. I hope I don't have to tell you why!

You don't want to offend your co-workers, so make sure these items are close enough to you that only you can smell them. Otherwise you could become labeled a challenging co-worker!

Sight

Using your sight to remind you of a special person, pet, vacation, or goal is an ideal way to help you relax. I mean, tell me a person who would not melt at the sight of a puppy with those sweet little eyes full of love and hope just staring back at you. Hang up an ideal vacation destination that will give you hope.

Make a Mini Vision Board

Design a mini vision board to place in a strategic place near your workspace that you can see often. If you are unfamiliar with what a vision board is, it is a collection of goals, ideas, pictures, affirmations, or sayings created to help you envision the life you want to have, things you want to acquire, or places you want to see. It's a way to visualize the way you want your life to be. A vision board encourages you to strive to be your best. If a vision board will cause you anxiety because you are not there yet, I would suggest you use another way to relax.

Name five things you would include in a vision board.

1. _____
2. _____
3. _____
4. _____
5. _____

Breathing

In my opinion, breathing is the beginning, middle, and ending of relaxation. When you can master breathing, specifically deep breathing, you are golden. We all know how to breathe. I mean, you wouldn't be reading this excellent and informative book if you couldn't breathe. But can you mindfully and deeply breathe? When you take deep breaths and slowly release, you activate that parasympathetic nervous system I was talking about earlier. This activates your calm mode. You can deep breathe for one minute and find some benefit. If you can do it longer, all the better.

Meditation

Meditation incorporates mindful breathing. What it does is train your mind to focus on a particular thing, idea, or vision to calm and focus your mind. In this, you gain better clarity and purpose.

There are different types of meditation, and I encourage you to learn about them and find the right fit for you.

Just like breathing, you can meditate virtually anywhere. You just need to sit comfortably.

Prayer

If you are religious, you are fully aware that prayer gives you a time to connect to your higher power. If this is a great way for you to destress, then do this. If it involves chants or sayings, you may need to do this in a more private area.

Stretches

Stretching those muscles involuntarily recruited in stressful and anxious moments can promote relaxation at work. Yes, you can do it at work, just sitting at your desk. If you don't work at a desk during the day, you can still stretch tense muscles. You can stretch in your car, when you using the restroom, in the cafeteria—pretty much anywhere.

Described below are a few stretches you can do.

(Note: Before you stretch, don't forget to either put in your earplugs for silence or your earphones with relaxing music. While you are at it, squirt a scent from your mister in the air and think of that puppy. It will make the experience, no matter how brief, enjoyable.)

Let's get started! Sitting with good posture, both feet on the floor, you can take a huge deep breath or even yawn, and as you exhale, drop your head to your chest or as far as it will go. Just let it hang. After 60 to 90 seconds, turn your head slightly in either direction, and use your hand to apply gentle traction to your head. Hold this for 60-90 seconds and then turn your head the other way. This stretch will relax the trapezius and neck muscles.

Another stretch for the upper body is to hold your head facing down in your hands, with your elbows on the desk. Make sure to remove your eyeglasses if you wear them. Take ten deep breaths. This will relax your neck muscles.

When you are done breathing, you should massage your temples, forehead, and chin. You can place your thumbs in the supraorbital and infraorbital notch and press and hold.

You can also stretch out the muscles of the head and face. You can put on hypoallergenic gloves and a drop of an essential oil the back of your hands so that when your hands are near your face, you can inhale that fragrance. Touch any area of your face and use a circular motion to move those facial muscles around.

To stretch the muscles of the neck, turn your head in all directions. Hold in position for 90 seconds.

Stand on a wall with your shoes on (or you can fall). Slowly lower yourself to an almost sitting position. This will loosen tight lower back muscles. You can also stretch your back by lifting up your leg and turning. You can use a towel to gain leverage.

Stretch your feet and ankles by rotating them in circular motions in both directions for 30 seconds each.

In 15 minutes or less, you can have a relaxed body.

It is important to hold these stretches for 90 seconds so the muscle fibers can relax and reset to a new relaxed point.

Posture

Sitting with good posture relaxes the tension in your lower back. Having your spine aligned as much as possible evenly distributes the pressure through the entire spine. When you are hunched over at your desk, your body weight puts pressure on your bones and joints and misaligns muscles. Good posture can help decrease physical stress.

Walking

Walking for relaxation can dissipate nervous energy or anxiety. Here, you are utilizing your major muscle groups and your lungs. You are increasing oxygenation to you brain and all body parts. Walking is also a great time for self-reflection. Benefits of walking are numerous. In the context of mindfulness, walking is beneficial in helping you calm your mind.

Journaling

Journaling is a mental and emotional release. When you are able to write something down, you can see it and it becomes more tangible. You are transferring your emotions and thoughts to another form. After you write something down, you have one of two things you can do. You can add to it and then self-reflect at a later time on how far you have come, or you can rip that piece of paper out, tear it up, or burn it. Either way, it is a release.

Affirmations

Affirmations are positive and conscious thoughts that you want to speak into existence in your life. You speak it from the ending, like its already there. You can write your affirmations on paper and place them where you can see them daily. You can constantly speak them. The idea is to replace negative and non-productive thoughts in your mind.

Things To Remember

Things To Remember

Things To Remember

Things To Remember

Chapter 10

DECLUTTER YOUR OFFICE SPACE

How do you feel when you walk in to an area and there is paper everywhere or there is no order or organization? Do you feel stressed and anxious when you see it? I do. Isn't it frustrating when you are rushing to find something and you can't find it where you think you last left it? You have papers, magazines, or reports on your desk or shelf that are three years old. Yes, I am speaking from personal experience. That was me. You just move stuff around on your desk, and before you know it, your desk is a pit of despair. Having a messy space is enough to make any person stressed out just looking at it.

You deserve to work in a well-organized space free from extra mind garbage so you can do your job effectively. You already have enough to deal with at work. Why add to it?

To declutter your office, you will need a few things.

A Determined and Positive Attitude

You will be adopting an attitude of release. Remember, let it go. Mindset is key when undertaking this endeavor. You must resolve within yourself that you are making a positive impression in your work life. My nurse was helping me trim down a stack of papers that I have literally not touched (unless it was to move to another area of my office to "get to" later) for three or four years! Wow! There was a point when I had tears in my eyes because this was such a monumental experience for me. I was literally letting go of a past that served me no purpose. I was sad to let it go and happy and relieved at the same time. When I have things on my desk that are starting to pile up, I see how decreasing or eliminating this stack brings my anxiety way down.

Even to this day, my wonderful nurses know when they walk by my office and see stuff on my desk to help me get it tamed down. It really does decrease my anxiety.

I challenge you to leave your workspace clean and organized each time you leave work for the day. When you arrive the next day, you will see a prepared space—a space that says "Yes, I am ready! Yes, I am organized! Yes, I am prepared!" It is so inspiring. You will no doubt feel alert and motivated. You can do this for you!

Time

If you need to come into work an hour early or leave an hour late temporarily, that's what you will need to do. If you need to come in over a weekend for a few hours, that's all the better. Even if you need to take a vacation day to come in and get things organized, do it! I will even go out on a limb and say yes, even if you are unpaid, it will be well worth it. The peace of mind and sense of calm that you will have when your space is decluttered is actually priceless.

A Few Tangible Things

You will need a shred box or folder, boxes or plastic bins depending on what you are separating, sticky notes, markers, folders in which to place important documents, storage organizers (to make your space look cute), a scanner, a camera or smartphone (be cognizant of taking photos with identifying information), and a trash can or garbage bags.

At the end of this book is a checklist you can copy and use to help you declutter your work/office space.

Make a list of what you want to declutter so that when you check each item off, you will feel accomplished and motivated to go to the next item. I started with my left desk drawer, then middle drawer, then right, then the table I had in the corner with papers. Break it down into little tasks.

What I Need to Declutter List

1. _____
2. _____
3. _____

4. _____

5. _____

You will need a dedicated helper who will keep you in check and tell it like it is. When you are wavering about whether you need to keep something, this person will be instrumental in having you keep things in perspective. For example, I once had one of my helpers ask me, "Dr. Gorman, do you really need this syllabus from that conference you went to four years ago?" Well, I guess I didn't. Your helper can be a spouse, child, coworker, or friend. Just make sure you have the clearance to have them in your private space, as it may contain confidential information. A non-employee may need to sign some type of document in order to be there. In the medical industry, there is HIPAA. You medical folks know what I'm talking about.

Having said that, you may have to be your own dedicated worker. Don't worry, you got this. No. *We* got this.

Please look in the back for a bonus checklist on ways to declutter your workspace.

You need to separate your things into five categories:

1. Things to throw away without having to think about it

    ▸ This will include wrappers, empty non-reusable containers, and old/expired snacks.

2. Things you can't live without

    ▶ If there was an emergency evacuation, this is what you would take.

3. Things you need to get to within the next two weeks

4. Thing you need to address now

5. Things you can give away that would give someone else some benefit

When you are thinking if you should keep something, ask yourself, "Will this help me perform better at work? Will this benefit me? What purpose will this serve? Will this increase my anxiety or decrease it?" If you know it will increase your anxiety, you know what to do with it. Throw it away.

Put that shredder and scanner to good use. If you truly don't need it, just release it!

Things To Remember

Things To Remember

Things To Remember

Things To Remember

Things To Remember

Chapter 11

ZEN YOUR WORK SPACE

Zen has taken on the meaning of relaxation, meditation, or being in a state of calm. What do I mean by "Zen your work space"? I am talking about creating a personal work atmosphere, no matter how big or small, because when you are in it, you feel calmer and more at peace. Yes, even at work. It can be, but it doesn't have to be anything elaborate or fancy. Just whatever makes you feel good and calm when you see it. Look at some magazines to get some ideas.

I want you to be able to create a "work home" on any budget. I am envisioning you coming to work and feeling an immediate sense of calm when you arrive into your office, cubicle, or workspace.

Here are some ways to "Zen your work space":

Post Positive, Inspirational, or Funny Sayings

You can think of something yourself or download things from the Internet. This would be a great time to place up a couple of those positive affirmations. Take a few moments to look online and find sayings that speak to you. Posting something up that makes you smile or laugh can be just as relaxing.

Zen Garden

Using a sand Zen garden is a physical way to destress. Using the rake to make sand waves, forming designs, or rearranging the stones can help take your mind off of stressors. A Zen garden adds to the relaxing atmosphere.

Running Water

Being a Pisces, water is my favorite element! For me, it represents a cleansing, a flow. Just looking at the ocean or even a running stream makes me feel the calmest. When I was younger, I would be reminded to turn the water off. But just hearing the water run made me feel better. I would also lose track of time when in the shower. Running water brings in the new and takes away the old. Having a little water fountain near you is not only very relaxing but also cathartic. I have a table top water fountain myself.

Live Plant(s)

Having something alive in your office or work space other than yourself is mandatory in my opinion. It represents hope, vitality, strength, and growth. It also livens up your work space. I have plants in my office, including bamboos. To me, a healthy plant just looks happy!

Lovely Pictures

Whatever you determine to be beautiful, calm, and nurturing, you should post. Of course, I would recommend it not be too controversial. Remember that more than likely, other people will see it, and this can invite negative comments, which can lead to arguments, which is—you got it—stressful.

Things To Remember

Things To Remember

Things To Remember

Things To Remember

Things To Remember

Chapter 12

SELF-CARE

This may be the most important chapter in this book because it's all about you. You are the most important person in your life whether or not you want to believe it or not. If you want to be the best at whatever you are doing, you need to be the best you. This means caring for yourself, loving yourself, and nourishing yourself. This means creating the time to do things, experience things, or partake in things that will bring you joy and inner peace.

Let me ask you—what is the cost of your life? Would you rather invest in being well or getting well?

Physical Self-Care

One form of physical self-care is getting regular massages.

Massages serve many purposes. They allow you to pamper yourself, relax your muscles, practice your deep breathing, "escape" from your hectic schedule, meditate, clear your mind, ease muscle pain, improve sleep, improve range of motion, increase flexibility, decrease depression and anxiety, improve circulation, lower blood pressure, reduce fatigue, improve digestion, improve your concentration, and stimulate lymph flow, thus improving your immunity. I mean really, why wouldn't you want this.

You'll also want to get regular checkups and health exams to make sure you are monitoring what you need to monitor. Prevention is the cornerstone of true health. This includes eye checkups and dental checkups.

Getting regular exercise is a cornerstone of physical self-care. Being more mobile and flexible and having better endurance and strength ensure your vitality. Being able to effectively use what you have will certify your self-confidence. When you are self-confident, you are free from the inside.

Lose weight if you are overweight. Just losing 10 percent of your body weight improves your overall health. There are numerous benefits to losing weight. Physically, being overweight places more physical stress on your joints and bones. We get into our eating habits, and I'll be the first one to admit, they are hard to get out of. But you have to ask yourself (and I had to ask myself) what benefit the extra weight is serving you. You may not figure this out in reading one book, but it needs to be addressed. So if you need to get counseling, get it. Join an online support group. Do what you need to do. You have only one body.

Mental Self-Care

Mental self-care is paramount in relieving stress. After all, how you deal with any adverse situations begins in your mind. How you perceive any situation will depend on your mindset. Two people can look at or experience the same thing, and one person can see it as a detriment while another person can see it as an opportunity to uplift himself. Which way are you viewing things?

Being able to express your feelings verbally and non-verbally will help you lighten your stress.

Nutritional Self-Care

Adequate hydration is key. All of our metabolic processes occur in water. Being well hydrated means that toxins are either flowing out of your body or nutrients are being delivered to your body. Hydration also promotes lubrication of our joints and tissues. Think of a plant that needs water. If you haven't watered it for a few days, it looks down and limp. After you water it and return the next day, it appears perky and vibrant. It works the same way with you. So take hydration seriously. Most experts recommend eight glasses of water per day.

Nutrition is the best. I know you have heard of the adage "You are what you eat." If you eat crap, you will feel like crap. Sure, it may taste good going down, but what comes of it? Diabetes, hypertension, or cancer. You already are stressed. Why add more to it? You need to feed your body with beneficial, nutritional foods with little to no processing, added hormones, chemicals, and pesticides so that your body will respond.

Spiritual Self-Care

Praying if you are religious, connecting to your higher power, or acknowledging something greater than yourself can help you acquire inner peace and thus destress. If you are not religious at all, this is fine too. Looking inside yourself for strength, clarity, and hope is all you need to connect. Please do this.

Social Self-Care

Being non-social can be just as beneficial as being social. Sometimes you want to be alone just to get your thoughts together or just or do something you want to do. For me, I just love taking the time to be alone in complete silence or listening to instrumental music. On the other hand, you may feel better being around that special person or people, and that's fine too, as long as it is relaxing for you. Taking time to "unplug" from social media or turning off your mobile phone even for a couple of hours can help you to relax. You can change your voicemail message to reflect that you are turning your phone off for a certain number of hours. I realize not having your phone turned on can cause extra stress for you, and if this is the case, at least place it on vibrate while you take this time for self-care.

Time Off

Please, please, please use your vacation days. They are designed to get you away from it all. This would be the ultimate time for you to destress. If you are not able to use all your vacation time, just use some of it. You need to take time away from work. Why not take a staycation? Let me tell you—sometimes time can be more valuable than money. I'm just saying. Spending quality time with your family or loved ones or even by yourself is something that you deserve. Use your sick days. Get your checks ups. Don't neglect yourself. In this case, *don't* let it go. Early detection of a lot of issues saves lives. That anxiety you are feeling could be an underlying thyroid condition in which your thyroid gland is overactive. This is treatable. Wouldn't it be something to learn that a big contributor to your stress and anxiety is because your thyroid gland is overactive?

Sleep

Get enough sleep. It is very difficult to have good focus and concentration if you are dozing. It's even worse if you are dozing off at work. Being sleep deprived causes poor memory, poor judgment, fatigue, body aches, and a sense of feeling off balance.

I remember sometimes when I was on call, I just couldn't think. I just couldn't get it together. I would actually doze off and have full dreams in a matter of a minute!

Sleep apnea is an underdiagnosed medical condition that has major health consequences. Sleep apnea occurs when the tissues and supporting muscles in the back of your neck and throat relax, occluding the free flow of air into and out of your lungs. Restful sleep is difficult to obtain when you are not breathing freely. You are not effectively exchanging oxygen. Your body has a way of waking you up to let you know you have to breathe. You may wake up feeling startled. That's your body telling you to wake up because it can't breathe!

There are two stages of the sleep cycle—non-REM (non-rapid eye movement) and REM (rapid eye movement). The stage of sleep you are in signifies to your brain when to rest and repair itself.

Not being able to have a restful night's sleep is not good. Being a doctor, I have spent so many nights with disrupted sleeping patterns. It shouldn't be considered normal for me but it is. I know there are many of you out there whose minds seems to never shut down when you are lying in bed anticipating sleep.

Some things you can try to help you get a good night's sleep include:

- Not drinking caffeinated beverages a few hours before you go to sleep
- Playing instrumental music in bed. You don't want to listen to music to which you may know the words, as you will spend your time singing instead of sleeping
- Taking a nice shower or bath to relax those stressed muscles. Use a relaxing body wash scent.
- Meditating or deep breathing in the bed
- Sipping a calm-prompting tea (but remember, it is water, and it can run right through you)
- Avoiding naps during the day if this is the cause of you not sleeping at night
- Avoiding alcohol
- Losing weight (this is one treatment for sleep apnea/snoring)
- Keeping the temperature of the room a little cool

I can't really advocate for the use of any particular medication in this forum because I believe in trying to naturally fall asleep, but if you are unable to, this is a discussion to have with your physician.

Make It Right at Home

In my opinion, home is supposed to be your ultimate place of calm and relaxation. The place you go to no matter what kind of day you are having to just be yourself. However, I realize there can be a lot of stress at home as well. You bring this stress to work. So you are stressed at work *and* at home. This is not good. If there are any issues at home that need to be addressed, do that. If you know there are areas of your home that stress you out when you look at them, fix them. Don't let arguments with your loved ones fester. A home should be a place of love, peace, and harmony. When you have a tough stressful day at work, the last thing you want is to go home and have more of the same, so make it right at home.

Name five ways you will practice self-care.

1. _____
2. _____
3. _____
4. _____
5. _____

Things To Remember

Things To Remember

Things To Remember

Things To Remember

Bonus

WORK STRESS ACTION PLAN

What is a work stress action plan? Well, have you heard of an action plan? An action plan is a set of strategies you can implement before something detrimental occurs. The best example I can give you is an asthma action plan. People with asthma who are undergoing an asthma attack must act quickly so that they can breathe. If they can't breathe, then they die.

Well, the same principle applies to the work setting. You can use an action plan.

I call it a work stress action plan because in times of immediate stress at work, you need to do something quickly before things get out of hand. You can intentionally deescalate a potentially devastating outburst or action. Haven't there been times at work where you want to yell at someone or do something even worse because you are just so angry or frustrated with a person or a situation? It's not good to be reactive in general. In the work setting, it can really be devastating. It can cause you to lose your job or even land you in jail.

It's unfortunate in our time that the stresses of work and life can lead to workplace violence. There is the potential for violence in the workplace in any place of employment. By no means is this work stress action plan that I am presenting a cure for mental illness, but in the immediate time, I feel there are a few strategies you can put to use to decrease the possibility of having a horrible outcome.

Follow these steps in order.

1. Be Quiet. Please don't talk, yell, or say anything. Your words are powerful. You can't take them back.

2. Smile.

3. Take deep breaths.

4. Talk with your higher power.

5. Recite your saying to calm down. My favorite thing to say is "It is what it is."

These things above can be done in one minute.

Other suggestions for your action plan are

1. Take a walk.

2. Go get a drink of water, juice, tea, or coffee. Avoid energy drinks. Of course, no alcohol.

3. Do some neck and back stretches.

4. Listen to familiar music that you love.
5. Use a physical de-stressor, like a squeeze ball, color, or sand garden.

I want you to list some other things that you can do that will allow you to immediately destress.

1. _____
2. _____
3. _____
4. _____
5. _____

Things To Remember

Things To Remember

Things To Remember

Things To Remember

Things To Remember

Bonus

A MESSAGE TO COMPANY HEADS, BUSINESS OWNERS, MANAGERS, AND BOSSES

Do you remember when you first started your company? Or better yet, do you remember when you were working for someone else? How did you feel at work? Were you stressed? If so, how would you have wanted to be treated. Now that you are charged with being the head, how do you want things to be? Do you want your employees to give their all? Do you want them to be loyal to you? How about productive? I truly believe that as the head, you set the culture of your company or business. Even if you are a manager, it is your obligation to get your juniors into action.

Being able manage different people with their different personalities, beliefs, educational backgrounds, and demeanors can be at the very least stressful. But you of all people understand the concept of the importance of working together to achieve a common goal if this is to be a profitable and beneficial business. You want satisfied stakeholders.

You have the power to change your company's "energy." You want your employees to make you money while you make your mark in your community or the world in a positive way.

In addition to being a doctor, I have always wanted to be a business owner. It's in my blood. Both of my parents were business owners. Some people say that it's easy to start a business, and I guess there may be a little truth to that. But I know it's hard to maintain a business. In my knowledge of business workings, I do know you need a plan. And I do understand that the cornerstone of any successful business is having employees who do their job well. I know how hard your employees will work for you is a reflection on how much you appreciate and cherish them.

Here are a few suggestions I believe will improve employee morale and foster a less stressed and more relaxed, productive work atmosphere.

Communication

Encouraging communication with your employees is key. There are many different ways to communicate. I know you are busy, but if some time can be made available for in-person employee interaction, this can be so great. When you are more informed about another person, you may find that there are more common points than differences. You can create a work family by getting to know one another.

Try to meet in person with small group of random employees. Let them know your story (I know you have one), and you hear theirs. Thank them for working for you. Make sure they are aware of your mission and core values.

Make sure your employees are well informed of changes in the company.

Employees need to be clear of what is expected of them when they come to work.

Encourage anonymous honest evaluations of your company and of employee supervisors, even if it's an independent company who does the surveys. Managers and supervisors need evaluations too.

When you pass an employee in the hall, say hello and acknowledge them. A brief moment is all it takes and can mean everything.

Encourage employee interactions on your time and on your dime. Have it during business hours, even if it's a couple of hours. You have a captive audience. Have self-improvement lectures, activities, classes, meet-and-greets, and snacks. Promote a dialogue with employees. Help them build positive relationships with each other.

Have a non-holiday themed "meet my family" night. Wear nametags. Let people see you are a real person.

Do Your Best to Accommodate Employee Schedules

Even though it may be hard to believe, employees do have lives outside of work (just a little sarcasm there)! Some are the heads of families, some have health problems, some are caregivers, some have children, and some may even have another job trying to make ends meet. Employees may have things that come up. Life happens, and it's not always outside of when they are supposed to be working.

I know it's not always possible depending on the job, but if possible, make the effort to hear your employee's request. If they have to veer a little off schedule to handle urgent personal matters, maybe its worth it. It's a kind gesture. Can you imaging the amount of loyalty you would have if your employee felt that you were in their corner?

Negotiate hours. Some people may have different out-of-work obligations and may need to work outside of normal business hours. They may need to work later or earlier or may not be able to work full days. If you can accommodate this, your employees will be appreciative and work harder when they are there and are likely be more productive.

Employee Praise

It's really excellent to acknowledge and praise employees who are top producers and earners for the company, and nothing is wrong with that. But what if you picked a random employee, no matter their work title, and recognized them as well? Highlight that they are important to your company.

Have a day where you cater lunch for no reason. Give that extra special touch and include foods for vegetarian, kosher, and gluten-free employees. Keep this information on file.

Recognize years of service by not only giving acknowledgement but also gifts or bonuses.

Establish an Employee Wellness Program

Do you have an employee well ness program? If you do, great for you! Maybe there is some room for improvement. Having healthier employees is beneficial all around. Consider adding to it by incorporating relaxation into it. Hire a consultant or speaker (hint hint) who can come into your business and give insight on how you can incorporate relaxation into your work principles (no matter how big or small) and educate your employees on the benefits of learning to relax and destress at work. Have classes on relaxation and how to better cope with stress at work. Remember that healthy (and happy) employees are more productive employees. More productivity equals more profits.

Create a Relaxation Room/Space

Have a room or partition of a room designated as a "relaxation zone" or "destress zone." Here, employees can come and take off their shoes and read, meditate, deep breathe, listen to music with their earphones, or just relax. This will be a safe zone free of any distractions. You can also create a "no talking zone" or "turn off cell phone zone." This would be a great place to come and destress during breaks. When it's time to get back to work, you are ready to go, recharged and relaxed. Bring in a company that will give on-site massages. Look for me to provide this service in the future.

Be Nice, Respectful, and Fair

Yes, I understand that it takes a certain grit, tough hide, thick skin, ambition, and confidence to run a business, but I personally believe you can be all those things and be nice to people.

Please don't criticize employees in front of others. Humiliation brings down morale. In my opinion, you can run a business, be professional, and still display integrity and compassion.

Last and certainly most, realize that just as much as your employees need you to earn a living, you need them to sustain a successful business. What kind of work atmosphere do you want to foster? If your child were working for someone, how would you want them to be treated by their boss? Having a healthy company to me means having healthy employees. Healthy employees work better, thrive, and produce more. Encourage that health by allowing them to deal with their stress.

Things To Remember

Things To Remember

Things To Remember

Things To Remember

Bonus

COLOR NOW (3 PAGES OF COLORING)

Coloring isn't just for children. It is a known and proven fact that coloring can decrease your stress and anxiety. It causes you to focus on the present while you are creating something beautiful. You portray positive thoughts. If you have never colored as an adult before, give it a try. You may like it. Use colored pencils or crayons. Turn on some nice music and color away!

Here I have added three coloring pages. Get to it!

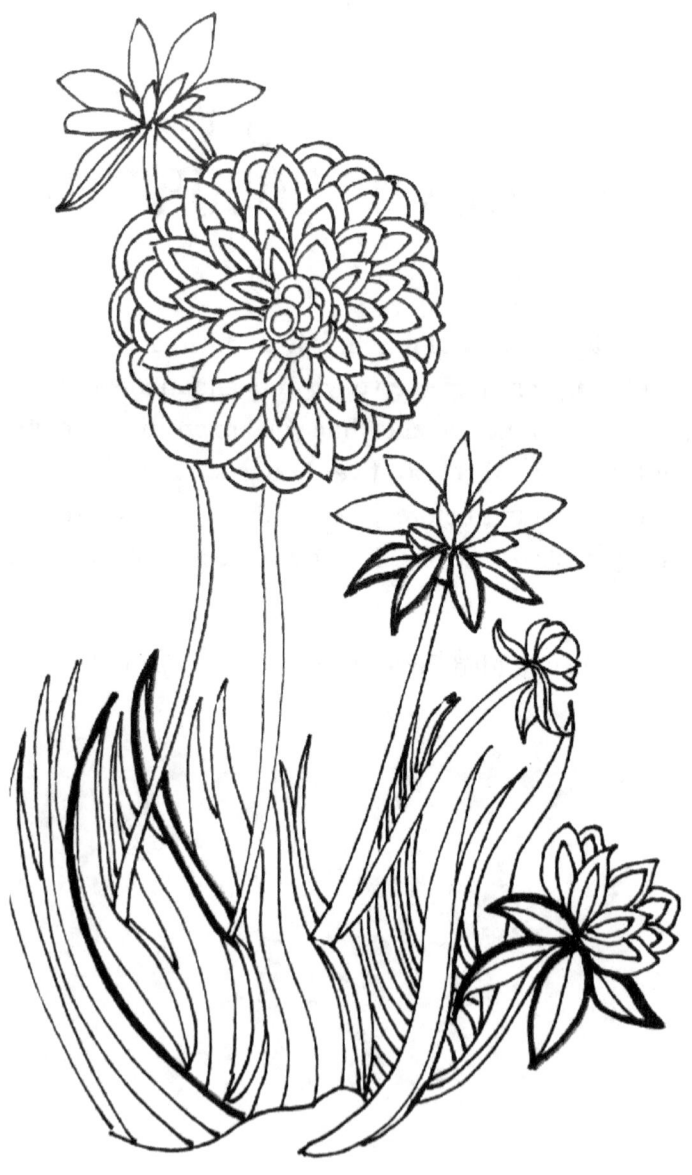

Relaxed and Ready

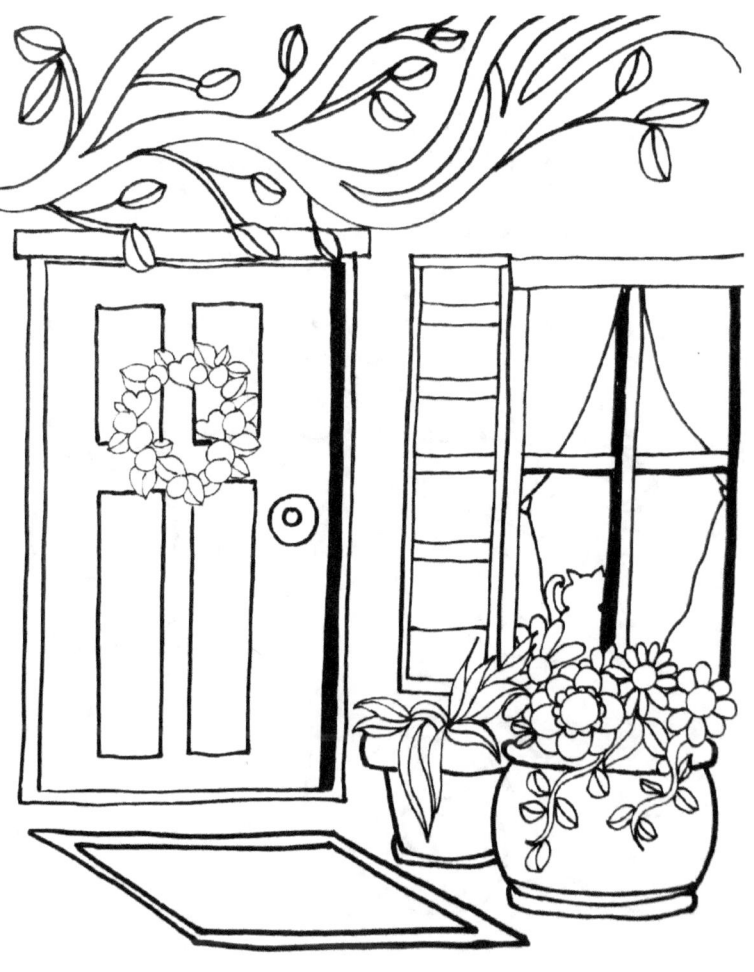

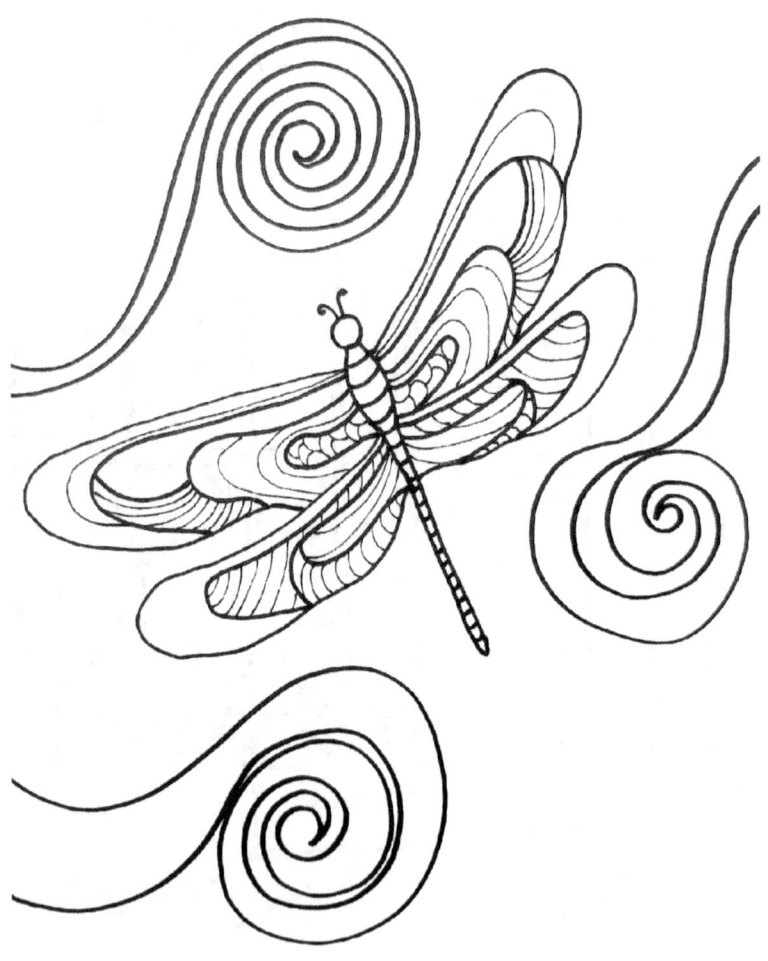

Bonus

30 DAYS OF CALM

A 30 Day Interactive Planner to Help You Destress at Work

Here, I have provided you 30 different things you can do every day at work that can help calm your mood or bring a little bit of joy to your life. Feel free to make copies and then check off the items each day. You can go out of order or do an item twice.

Note that a lot of these may need to be done during your lunch break when you may have more time.

DAY 1 ☐	DAY 2 ☐	DAY 3 ☐	DAY 4 ☐	DAY 5 ☐
Play your favorite song or listen to your favorite group from when you were in high school during your lunch time	Start your work space vision board, day one of three	Meditate (imagery)	Eat not one but two pieces of dark chocolate while listening to music	Sit outside in the sun for 15 min and deep breathe
DAY 6 ☐	**DAY 7** ☐	**DAY 8** ☐	**DAY 9** ☐	**DAY 10** ☐
Get a manicure, pedicure, or massage	Take a 30-minute nap (be sure to set your alarm!)	Work on day two of three on your work space vision board	Hand write a thank you note or thinking of you note	Put on your office footies and do stretches
DAY 11 ☐	**DAY 12** ☐	**DAY 13** ☐	**DAY 14** ☐	**DAY 15** ☐
Shout out your work frustrations in your car (with the windows rolled up)	Watch videos on your phone of puppies / kittens playing	Take 10 deep breaths while visualizing a happy thought	Eat your favorite lunch	Watch something really funny on your phone
DAY 16 ☐	**DAY 17** ☐	**DAY 18** ☐	**DAY 19** ☐	**DAY 20** ☐
Get a temple and scalp massage	Color	Go for a walk while listening to your favorite music	Read a favorite magazine or chapter of a book	Complete day three of three of your vision board

DAY 21 ⬜	DAY 22 ⬜	DAY 23 ⬜	DAY 24 ⬜	DAY 25 ⬜
Use an essential oil breathing mask	Search online for vacation destinations	Call your best friend and see what they are up to (at lunch time)	Leave your work premises for a walk	Wash your hands in warm water with scented soap and use scented hand lotion after you dry
DAY 26 ⬜	**DAY 27** ⬜	**DAY 28** ⬜	**DAY 29** ⬜	**DAY 30** ⬜
Take your besties out to lunch	Make designs on your sand garden	Use a stress release toy like a stress ball or a twirler	Put a plant on your desk and name it	Get a chair massage or foot massage

Thank you very much for reading my book.

What can I say about stress? I have it. You have it. We all have it. Will it ever leave? Nope. Can we learn to deal with it constructively so that it doesn't kill us? Absolutely. Even if you don't agree with all of the things presented in this book, that's okay. Try something presented here to help you become a better, more "relaxed and ready" you.

EXTRA STUFF

Log onto Facebook and request to join my closed group: The Relaxation Room with Dr. Deitrick. Become a "Zenie." Here, we will exchange ideas on how to relax. You will also get updates on where I will be appearing and be able to find out firsthand.

> Visit my websites:
>
> **www.DrDeitrickG.com**
> or
> **www.relaxedwithdrdeitrick.com**
>
> - Book me to speak at your company, organizational meeting, or conference
>
> - Subscribe to my blogs
>
> - View my webinars
>
> - Listen to my podcasts

MY DECLUTTER CHECKLIST

_____ Good Attitude/Release It Attitude (First and foremost. Check it twice!!)

_____ Scanner (To scan important documents)

_____ Shredder (After you scan, you can shred. You can also just shred what you don't need)

_____ Wet Wipes (Or the like to clean)

_____ Camera/Camera Phone (To take before and after photos and photos of important personal things you need to have readily accessible)

_____ Sticky Notes (To label stuff)

_____ Helper (If possible, to help you keep it real. Please remember confidentiality issues.)

_____ Boxes or Folders (To organize)

_____ Markers/Pens

_____ Storage Container

_____ Organizer

_____ Trash Bags/Cans

PRODUCTS COMING SOON

Check the website for:

- Personal Space Mister
- Essential Oils
- Relaxation Mask
- "Work in Zen" Relaxation Box
- Adult Coloring Books
- T-Shirts
- Mugs
- 12-Month Calendar
- Other products

ACKNOWLEDGMENTS

Paula Mould, Illustrator, www.paulamould.com

Nurse Eva Sorrells, Model for Body Landmarks

Katrina Gorman, of Katrina Gorman Designs,
contact to provide original art and accessories to calm your office at www.katrinagormandesigns.com

REFERENCES

I dusted off a couple of medical school books to refresh:

1. *Atlas of Human Anatomy* by Frank Netter, MD, 3rd edition

2. *Principles of Physiology* by Robert M. Berne and Matthew N. Levy 3rd edition

3. *Physiology* by Linda S. Costanzo

I also took a look at www.endocrinology.org.

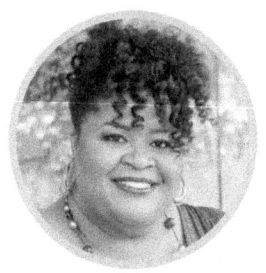

ABOUT THE AUTHOR

Dr. Deitrick Gorman is a board-certified family medicine practitioner whose lifelong dream was to become a doctor and a business owner. She has her Bachelor of Science from Purdue University, where she was part of the Zeta Phi Beta sorority; her Master of Science from Indiana University; and her doctorate from Rowan University. Her personal mission is to inspire professionals who find themselves stressed and unproductive to calm themselves so that they can be their best personally and professionally.

A resident of Pecos, Texas, Dr. Gorman enjoys traveling, listening to music, and collecting pencils. She is currently working on a coloring book for adults.

Learn more at www.DrDeitrickG.com

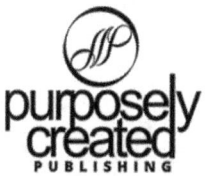

CREATING DISTINCTIVE BOOKS
WITH INTENTIONAL RESULTS

We're a collaborative group of creative masterminds with a mission to produce high-quality books to position you for monumental success in the marketplace.

Our professional team of writers, editors, designers, and marketing strategists work closely together to ensure that every detail of your book is a clear representation of the message in your writing.

Want to know more?
Write to us at info@publishyourgift.com
or call (888) 949-6228

Discover great books, exclusive offers, and more at
www.PublishYourGift.com

Connect with us on social media

@publishyourgift

www.ingramcontent.com/pod-product-compliance
Lightning Source LLC
LaVergne TN
LVHW021714060526
838200LV00050B/2655